THE TOTAL ME-TOX

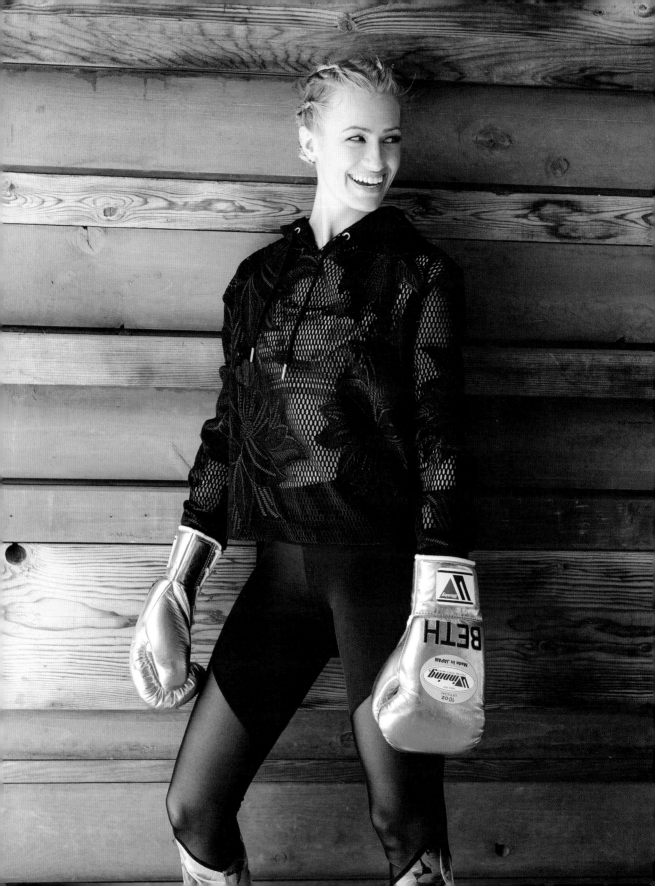

THE
TOTAL
ME-TOX

How to Ditch Your Diet,
Move Your Body & Love Your Life

BETH BEHRS

WITH WENDY SHANKER

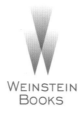

WEINSTEIN
BOOKS

Cataloging-in-Publication data for this book is available from the Library of Congress.

ISBN: 978-1-60286-308-8 (print)
ISBN: 978-1-60286-309-5 (e-book)

Published by Weinstein Books,
an imprint of Perseus Books, LLC,
a subsidiary of Hachette Book Group, Inc.
www.weinsteinbooks.com

Weinstein Books are available at special discounts for bulk purchases in the U.S. by corporations, institutions, and other organizations. For more information, please contact the Special Markets Department at the Perseus Books Group, 2300 Chestnut Street, Suite 200, Philadelphia, PA 19103, call (800) 810-4145, ext. 5000, or e-mail special.markets@perseusbooks.com.

First edition

10 9 8 7 6 5 4 3 2 1

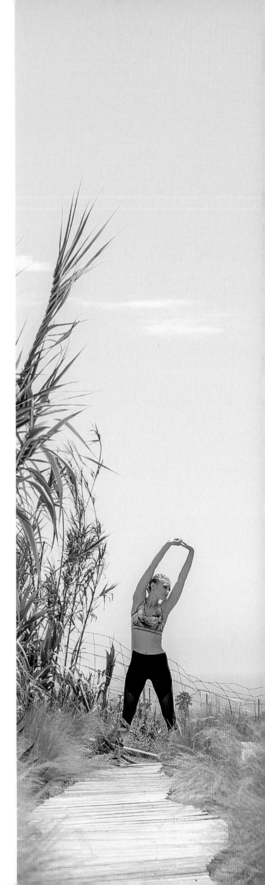

To Grammy. Who won't drink "the green sludge."
Love you bushels.

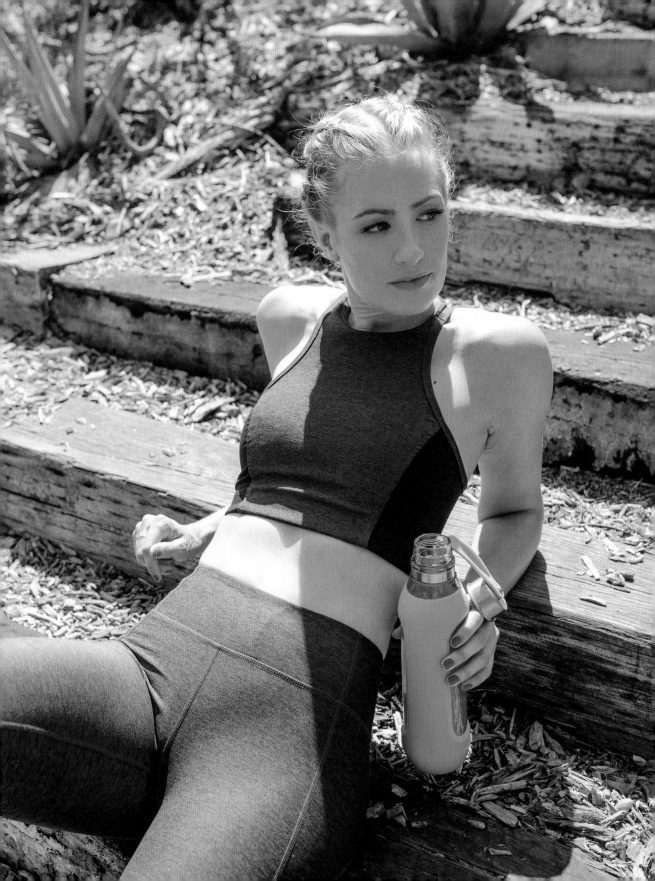

CONTENTS

Once we believe in ourselves,
we can risk curiosity, wonder, spontaneous delight,
or any experience that reveals the human spirit.

—E. E. Cummings

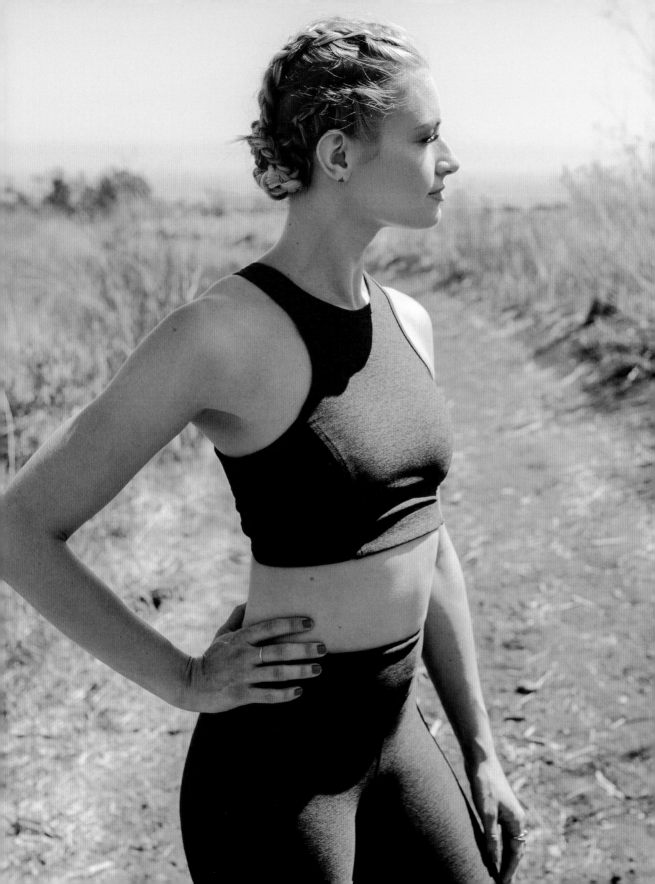

HI, YOU!

I'm so happy and honored that you're reading this book! See, I'm a lot of things: a performer, a singer, a passionate-if-clumsy dancer, a daughter, a sister, a friend, a homeowner, a soon-to-be wife, an activist, a good-health enthusiast, and an Etsy junkie. But I have never considered myself an author.

For me, writing is similar to most other experiences in my life—challenging, terrifying, exhilarating, and requiring a $#*!load of hard work. I've had several incredible, amazing years starring on *2 Broke Girls* on CBS, collaborating with some of the most talented people in the world . . . but it took years of blood, sweat, and tears (along with plenty of unanswered letters and phone calls) to get here. Let me bust a Hollywood (or Anywhere-wood) myth for you: Nothing happens overnight. The term "overnight sensation" should be banished from our vocabulary because it doesn't exist. (So should the words "moist" and "panties" . . . especially when they are used together.)

In my experience, uber-successful people have one thing in common: They work their freakin' *asses* off. Not just in their professional lives, but in their personal lives, too. By my definition, true success is more than making a lot of money. Or doing work you love but struggling to survive financially. It's having the respect of others and having respect for yourself. That takes passion, confidence, ingenuity, and encouragement. You need to make the most out of the time you have in your day. And you have to keep your body and mind steel-strong.

So while I may still be an author-in-training, I can definitely tell you a thing or two (or fourteen chapters' worth) about that last bit—keeping your mind, body, and spirit super strong—because I've put all kinds of intense work into earning my healthy-living stripes. I can offer you some really hard-won advice about how I went from being a motivated-yet-lazy sludge monster to being an active, healthy, energetic human being.

My journey began when I was in the middle of a full-on physical and mental crisis that required a complete detox to get to the other side. As I tried other people's plans and recommendations, I realized that in order to meet my goals, I had to clear my system on my own terms. What I needed was a ME-tox, not a detox.

Too many of us don't invest in our well-being until it's too late. We tell ourselves that we're not the priority, that we'll fix the problem later, or that our health isn't as important as our careers or relationships. But the truth is that you can't have a successful career or relationship if you're stuck in an unsuccessful body. You have to be in good health to go out and win the other challenges in your life. Realizing this was a revelation for me. In a weird way, I was *lucky* that my body literally broke down and rebelled against the way I was living. I had no choice but to take action. But while I knew I needed to make changes, I didn't want to compromise my happiness for the sake of my health. So I created my own path. And now, luckily, you can learn from my experience—without having to wait for your mind and body to suffer. Take control of your life TODAY.

On the pages that follow, I'll tell you about changes that I made to my diet (formerly all crap), workout routine (formerly nonexistent), and mental health (formerly a relentless state of panic and anxiety) that resulted in a much higher quality of life—and contributed to success in my career and relationships. I also feel connected to myself and my body in a way that I thought only monks, yoga teachers, and Kate Hudson were entitled to. I'd like to share that story with you because I know it's something we all aspire to. And it's a very worthy, very achievable aspiration. I'm still a work in progress (I think everyone is), but I love the idea of working *together* to—well, not to get all Oprah on you, but—be our best selves.

Before we get started, I'd like to tell you where I came from. When I was twenty-one years old, I was a semi-starving actor living in LA—yet somehow still eating crappy food and waaaay too much of it!—making about $400 a week nannying and doing humiliating personal-assistant jobs here and there. Good health was my lowest priority. My rent was $800 a month, so I shared a room with Courtney, one of my best friends from UCLA theater school. We had met junior year doing a Tony Kushner play together. (I'll admit, we were also doing a shot or two of tequila backstage to pass the time during tech rehearsals . . . so professional.) Courtney's side of the closet-size room was always immaculate, while mine looked like something out of *Grey Gardens*. We didn't live in the greatest neighborhood, and when a break-in happened right next to us, I put pots and pans by our door as an alarm—so if someone busted in, I could wake up and use my phone to call 911. (And maybe bash the burglar over the head with a frying pan?) I had no real social life . . . just my nanny job, the occasional audition, and no gas in my 1991 Mercury Mystique, which I had purchased from an old lady for $1,000. Money was tight—Spanx tight. So I wasn't going to spend it on useless stuff like gym memberships and fresh kale. But I refused to give up on my dream of success.

I had always known I wanted to be an actor. According to my parents, I was a toddler who loved acting out "So Long, Farewell" from *The Sound of Music* up and down our stairs every night. By the time I was in kindergarten, I was in theater. I can't remember a time when I wasn't connected to it.

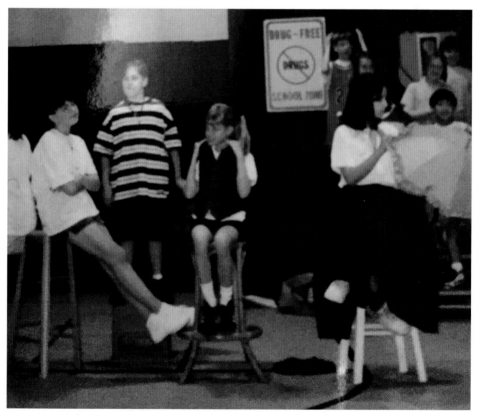

One of my first gigs: educational theater, playing *Jeopardy!* to show kids the dangers of drug abuse. "I'll take 'Listen to a seven-year-old talk about angel dust' for $1,000, Alex."

I landed my first play at the age of five—as a cat in *Snow White*—with one line. As I busted it out—something like, "No one will know it's the queen!" (How do I still remember that??)—I knocked over a table on the set. The audience thought I was hilarious. This was the beginning of my love for performing, and my complete inability to not be a total klutz while doing it. I've made an entire career in comedy based on facing my "truth" and embracing my flaws. My complete lack of grace turned into a natural ability to take pratfalls on a sitcom.

There were a few early signs that not just performance, but *comedy* performance, was what I really wanted to do. When I was in fifth grade, we had to do projects about explorers. I was assigned Ferdinand Magellan, the Portuguese explorer famed for organizing the Spanish expedition that eventually circled the globe. I came to school dressed as Magellan, doing a flamboyant version of him tripping over chairs and desks, pretending to circumnavigate the classroom. I had my class ROFL-ing all over the place. My teacher told people about it, and it got on the news. Seriously, in Lynchburg, Virginia, in 1996, a nine-year-old dressed as a Portuguese explorer doing bits about sixteenth-century Spain was newsworthy stuff.

My parents were educators, and my family moved a lot—Lancaster to Lynchburg to California—but I stayed in theater no matter where we were. I started

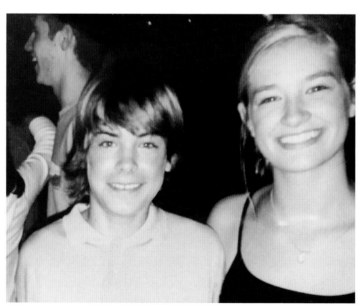

Look who went to acting camp with me! Even at thirteen, all the girls had crushes on little Zac Efron.

going to summertime acting camp when I was in kindergarten. When I was sixteen, I landed the role of Maria in an acclaimed local production of *The Sound of Music*. (Those nightly "auf wiedersehens" on my family's staircase really paid off!)

When I was a high school sophomore in 2001, we moved to Marin in Northern California. When I first walked into school, I was in shock: Pretty much the whole campus was outside, which was very different from my school in Virginia. The day I arrived, there was a schoolwide anti–Iraq War protest. The students were gathered on a big hill under a clock tower, ordering drivers to "Honk for peace!" I did not see a lot of that kind of thing in Lynchburg. Marin was a total contrast: really hippie-dippie, all Birkenstocks and pajama pants.

As I struggled to fit in, I turned to the love that had always sustained me: performing. I joined a theater group where the seniors directed the underclassmen. During warm-ups, we'd go around the room and share a good thing and a bad thing that was going on in our lives. One day I mentioned that eating lunch alone was pretty thorny for me. A junior named Meghan was horrified: "Today, you're eating with us!" A circle of friends was born, along with the knowledge that acting (and being around actors) was always going to be my happy place.

It was a risky call, but I decided to pursue acting as a career. I enrolled in theater school in Los Angeles, at UCLA. I started college as a musical theater major, which meant I had to take dance class for three hours a day. I quickly discovered that I didn't have the abilities that other students did. My skinny, semi-athletic body wasn't going to bump and grind like everyone else's—to this day, I dance to my own mildly uncoordinated drumbeat. Still, I gave it my all because that's all you can ever do! Today I use those skills every time I have to trip and fall and swoon and stumble on *2 Broke Girls*. (And despite my sucking at it, I do love to dance. Just the other night I was cooking dinner and had on an old Cole Porter/Ella Fitzgerald record. I was dancing by myself, making some chicken saagwala and brown rice [page 111]. Glad my Snapchat is gone in ten seconds!)

I had started auditioning for films and TV in college, but I wasn't getting a lot of acting jobs. It was the classic Hollywood Catch-22: If you don't have a résumé, you need jobs . . . but you need jobs to build a résumé. I was doing three auditions a month, and it was a really tough time. I didn't think about my health or well-being at all; it was a lot of mac and cheese and rushing around. I had a terrible job at a "high class" Mexican version of Hooters on the Sunset Strip. I quit because I didn't want to wear the referee uniforms assigned to the waitresses.

But, as they always say, the night is darkest before the dawn. I got a job working at the Geffen Playhouse, an amazing not-for-profit theater near UCLA. The Geffen was originally a Masonic lodge built in 1929. It has a very warm, country-house kind of vibe, in contrast to many of the sterile, modern theaters you see today. I started as an usher and then moved up to concierge, running the front desk and doing a little personal-assistant work here and there. Finally, I started bartending, a cool gig to get at the Geffen. I was hardly Tom Cruise in *Cocktail*, but I did make a mean gin and tonic.

Working at the Geffen was also a decent way for me to score auditions. For example, Alicia Silverstone needed an understudy in a new play they were doing there. So the casting agents called me and said I had an audition the next day. I was floored. The next morning I was on my way from the Palisades to Brentwood when, for whatever reason, traffic stopped dead—like rigor mortis dead. I watched the minutes tick by, knowing I was going to miss my slot. You have to understand: I'm never late. I'm early. (Being on time, if not early, is my professional law.) To this day I'm the earliest person on the set of *2 Broke Girls*. But that day, I ran into the Geffen sobbing because I knew I was so late. The director had left already.

A woman who was there must have taken pity on me—or maybe she could tell I had some talent under my smeared mascara—and said, "Oh, we are casting *American Pie* and you have to come by!" I blub-blubbered an acceptance to her invitation, trying to put on a brave front. On the way home I cried so much that I hit my car against a pillar in the parking garage, racking up like $10,000 of damage. It was one of those days—one of those months, years. (I couldn't afford to get the damage fixed until I landed *2 Broke Girls* three and a half years later.)

Wait, I was starting to say that something good happened. Oh yeah—I got the job! *American Pie*! Okay, so it wasn't the original *American Pie*, starring Jason Biggs with his you-know-what in a baked good and my now-good-friend Jennifer Coolidge in her legendary performance as "Stifler's mom." This was more like the seventh production in the series: *American Pie Presents: The Book of Love*. Straight to DVD. But it gave me the opportunity to work in Vancouver for three months with a bunch of twenty-one-year-olds and make a movie. It was the first time I had money, and we stayed in a five-star hotel. I played a virgin named Heidi, and I was the only girl who kept her clothes on in the whole movie. The people I met on that shoot are still some of my best friends.

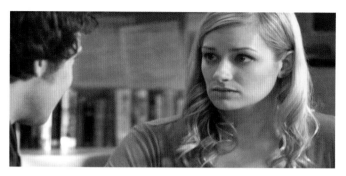

I played Maria in *The Sound of Music*, Sandy in *Grease*, and now Heidi in *Book of Love* . . . wow, I really got pigeonholed as a virgin for a while.

After the shoot I was consumed with getting more auditions. I went back to working at the Geffen and had a lot of fun. I loved my coworkers, including Adam, who was in my year at UCLA. (Side note: Adam is now a hand model. Seriously. He has hand shots and everything. He wore gloves bartending and got way more manicures than I ever did.) I met some amazing people who came through the Geffen, including the legendary Joan Rivers. She was doing a one-woman show, and I was thrilled to be chosen to run lines with her. She was like a grandma to me, and so generous. When Joan was getting a manicure, she'd offer to get me one, too (Adam was quite jealous). And she let me pick out pieces from her QVC jewelry line. I helped her go over her material every day, and she made me eggs. She remains one of my comedy heroes.

Besides working at the Geffen, I did a bunch of odd personal-assistant jobs, like scheduling and dog-walking and occasionally lugging giant jugs of Tide out of Costco and spilling them all over the parking lot. I also still nannied. I was burning the candle at both ends—which was hard because I could barely afford to buy candles. At night, the Geffen gang would get together and let off steam with the help of many, many bottles of wine. I woke up with a lot of hangovers back in those days. Plus, I couldn't seem to book acting jobs for the life of me.

One day Adam and I heard NBC was going to cast new interns on *The Office*. We decided to take power into our own hands, writing an *Office* parody and filming it at the Geffen. We played two very adversarial and not-too-bright friends who make a video audition to become interns at the Dunder Mifflin paper company in Scranton, Pennsylvania. In the seven-minute video, Adam and I alternately had each other's backs and were at each other's throats. He was clearly in love with me, and I was clearly hitting on the camera man (me purring, "I don't think I've ever seen eyes that chocolate brown!").

To our shock and delight, the video went viral and made it to the front page of the website Funny or Die! In the Internet comedy world, that's like getting your freakin' face on the cover of *Time* magazine. My agent was then able to send the tape out to casting directors. (While I'm going to offer you a lot of wellness advice in the pages that follow, let that be a career lesson to you: Don't wait for someone else to create success for you. Do it yourself!)

When the producers who were developing a new CBS comedy called *2 Broke Girls* saw the tape, they asked me to come in for an audition. The show was about two young women living together in Brooklyn, working at a diner. One of them, Max, was broke and always had been; the other, Caroline (the part I was after), was a trust-funder whose family had lost everything after her dad ended up in jail. The script was hilarious, and there were a lot of similarities between me and Caroline—mostly a sense of wounded-yet-rosy optimism. Caroline had a pink can of pepper spray and I did, too. The part was amazing—just too good to be true.

I was the first person to read for Caroline. It was 10 a.m. on a Thursday morning. I wore the same thing I wore to every audition: jeans I'd nipped from the set of *American Pie*, a super-flowy fancy-pants white blouse that my mom bought me for Christmas, and Frye cowboy boots. They were the only non-tomboy clothes that I had. I thought the audition went well, and I was pretty sure I would get a callback. I felt weirdly calm, like, *It's all going to be okay.* I've never again had that feeling after an audition. That was it: *This is going to be okay.* And a little: *No, it can't be, they're going to go with a big name.* But not too much of that! (The casting director, Julie, later told me that she went home that night and showed her family the reel, telling them, "I think I found the girl!") Sometimes you know when something works.

Then came a bunch of callbacks, where I read for the part over and over, getting a better take on Caroline each time. The process was intimidating, but I'd already met the incredible showrunner Michael Patrick King (I was in awe of his renowned talent on *Sex and the City*, one of my favorite shows ever) and cocreator Whitney Cummings, whom I loved on *Chelsea Lately*, Comedy Central roasts, and her own sitcom, *Whitney*. I kept telling myself, *If all else fails, at least I got to meet these creative people!*

When I got to the level where I was auditioning for the network, Michael Patrick King told me, "Beth, you *need* to get a pair of heels." (It was the first time—and not the last—that he took me under his wing.) I didn't have any heels. My shoe wardrobe consisted of a couple of pairs of California surf sandals, and when it got cold, I would wear my cowboy boots with skirts and jeans. If you watch the show (and I hope you do!), you know that Caroline is in pajamas and heels. Not wussy little kitten heels, but five- or six-inchers that make you stomp like a Victoria's Secret angel on the runway. I didn't own a thing that looked Upper East Side, let alone screamed it (i.e., Lululemon yoga pants, Burberry puffer coat, Givenchy boots, giant Birkin bag, and Tom Ford shades, natch), so I went to Nordstrom and bought a pair of simple black Steve Madden suede heels for about $200. I thought they were *very* high-end at the time—then again, I knew more about acting than fashion. But I stomped around confidently in my new shoes, hoping the next time I appeared in front of the network execs they'd give me the onceover and say, "There she is! There's our Caroline."

Those heels must have done the trick. After six auditions—six times trying to make stoic people laugh at lines they'd heard a thousand times, six times waiting for hours, sitting in a room chatting politely with girls who you know are your direct competition—CBS asked me to read with Kat Dennings. Kat had starred in movies like *The 40-Year-Old Virgin* and *Nick & Norah's Infinite Playlist*; she was already cast as Max. She was shooting a movie, but she flew to LA for an hour to do the audition with me. That was the moment everybody—even the two of us—thought, "Oh, hell yes! Let's do this!"

Kat was amazing. It's not often that you read with somebody and have this incredible chemistry. Honestly, I don't know if I will ever have that again with anyone. Now, years later, it's beyond acting chemistry. Beyond being good friends. Beyond being sisters, even. At that moment, after the final audition, I remember Kat looking at me in the elevator and saying, "Call me if it's not you because if it's not, I'm pulling out." An hour later they told me I got it. It was the best day of my life (so far). I will never forget it.

And now, we have so many seasons under our belt that we're in syndication. Crazy! We have a ridiculously good time shooting this show. I love the feeling of jumping off the plank with a joke, especially when we get a monologue ten minutes before we have to say it in front of a live audience . . . it's a ton of fear and adrenaline. When the joke lands and it does well, it's the greatest high in the

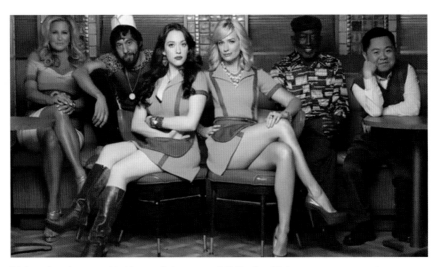
Living the dream with Kat and the cast of *2 Broke Girls*.

world, like you just shot up with heroin or something. (Not that I know. The craziest drug I've ever done is a $1 bottle of Champagne.)

I truly have the world's most amazing job. But it's not all easy-peasy. Shoot days are long, and when you're doing as much physical comedy as I am, it's an endurance contest. I quickly realized that I had to stay in shape, as on any given shoot day I might get thrown into a dryer and end up with bruises all up and down my back. That's not even a hypothetical; a stuntwoman, who was a roller derby girl in real life, threw me in an industrial dryer when we did a scene in a clothing factory. I got battle wounds. (Luckily, I also have amazing stunt coordinators.)

As Caroline, I've been flung into a dumpster; walked on a ledge in hail and rain while wearing seven-inch heels; rock climbed in stilettoes; got rope burn doing a striptease (don't ask); slipped on pearls; been wedged in a window while a Rottweiler licked baby food off my face; had my hair caught in a Murphy bed; and been tossed into a giant present by an elf while working at Santa Land. Poor hair and makeup department, God love 'em; I'm quite the cleanup on aisle two. But I had to bring my physical game up to my theatrical game—not just to survive each week of shooting, but to manage my body as it spiraled out of control. I quickly felt exhausted, burnt out, and depressed. I was in pain all the time. My skin started to turn dry, crusty, and scaly. My period stopped and my panic attacks—which had started freshman year of college after a horrible flight to New

York required an emergency landing—kicked up a notch. It got harder and harder to do what came naturally to me.

I bet you're going: "Yup, same here." You don't have to work on a TV show to feel the same way I felt. Maybe you're exhausted by your office job and feeling like only intravenous caramel cappuccinos will keep you going. Maybe the emotional roller coaster of working and mom-ing at the same time leaves you feeling—possibly more frequently than you'd like to admit—like leaving your kid in a parking lot (aw, you'll come back and get him soon, I'm sure!). Maybe your menstrual cycle is less cyclical and more Cirque du Soleil. Maybe your friends have convinced you to try some crazy diet—the Only Fish with Scales Diet, the All-Kiwi Diet, the Eat like a T-Rex Diet—and you are debating whether to throttle an innocent passerby snacking on a yogurt raisin.

You're not alone. And you can change it. After all, I did. It wasn't fast, and it wasn't easy . . . but I figured out how to ME-tox! I did it my own way, a lasting way.

I don't claim to have all the answers. But because I always wish I knew then what I know now, I want to help you avoid some of the missteps I made and give you the kick in the ass you need to help you get on top of your game. Sharing ideas and experiences helps us all to learn, grow, and evolve into the best versions of ourselves we can possibly be. I know for me it's important to feel like I'm not *alone* when I'm trying to make changes in my life, especially physical ones. That feeling of support—even when it's from people I don't know well—is what has gotten me through the toughest times and the biggest challenges in my life.

So this book is for all the fabulous people on Instagram and Twitter (yes, I see you!) who write me asking which recipes I use or what my favorite yoga poses are (and even, "*When the F* are you ever going to take off those pearls as Caroline Channing?" Answer: Never!). But you also ask me for advice on those days when you hate your body, how to make it to rent day with nothing in your pocket, and how to have hard conversations with people you care about. I hope I can provide some helpful answers in these pages—because I've been in every one of those situations more times than I'd like to admit. No secrets and no shame here! I'm hoping that if you hear what I went through and feel what I felt, then maybe you'll realize that there's a perfect place for you in this world and that there's a way to get there—without giving up on things that make you happy, like a sweet treat or a Stella. You can bring movement into your life without spending hours on a treadmill. You can find peace of mind without twisting yourself into a pretzel and wearing a robe.

I've had the phenomenal good fortune of crossing paths with people who have not only shown me ways to find power in feeling healthy and strong inside and out but who have inspired me to try harder, aim higher, and dream bigger than I ever thought I could. They have shown me how to believe in myself, and in turn have given me the opportunity to see the beauty, talent, and unique spirit in everyone I meet.

Including YOU.

It won't happen overnight—no overnight sensations, remember?—but little by little, bit by bit, smoothie by smoothie (I love smoothies), you can achieve your own image of success. And enjoy the process of getting it! You're going to do a ME-tox, not a detox. Well, a YOU-tox. You know what I mean! In the following pages, you'll find tips on physical and mental health, on spiritual centeredness, on beauty and self-confidence—from a person who used to live on doughnuts and pizza and thrive on stress. I believe following these tips and strategies will make you feel good and help lead you to the most joy possible. And that's what each and every one of us deserves.

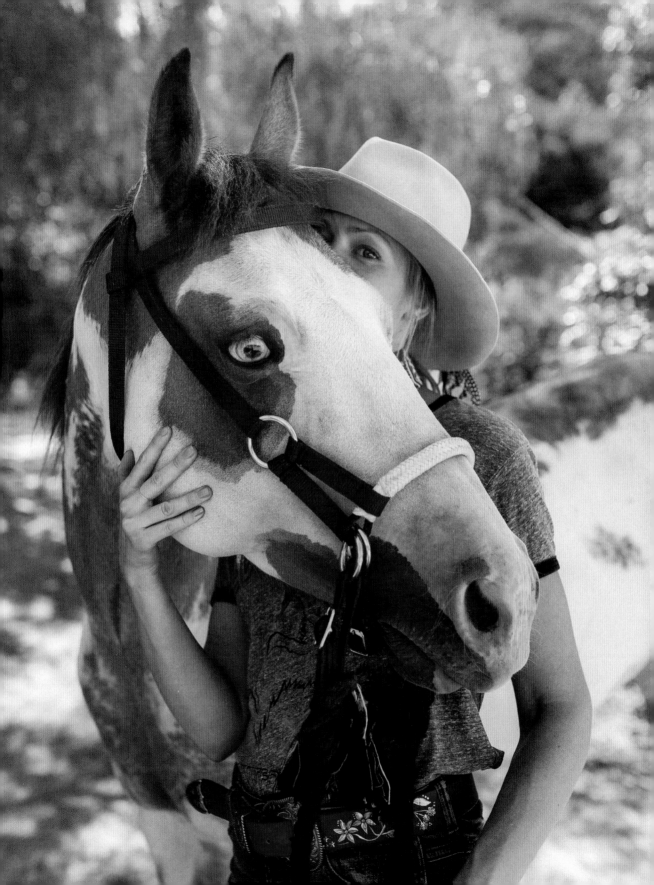

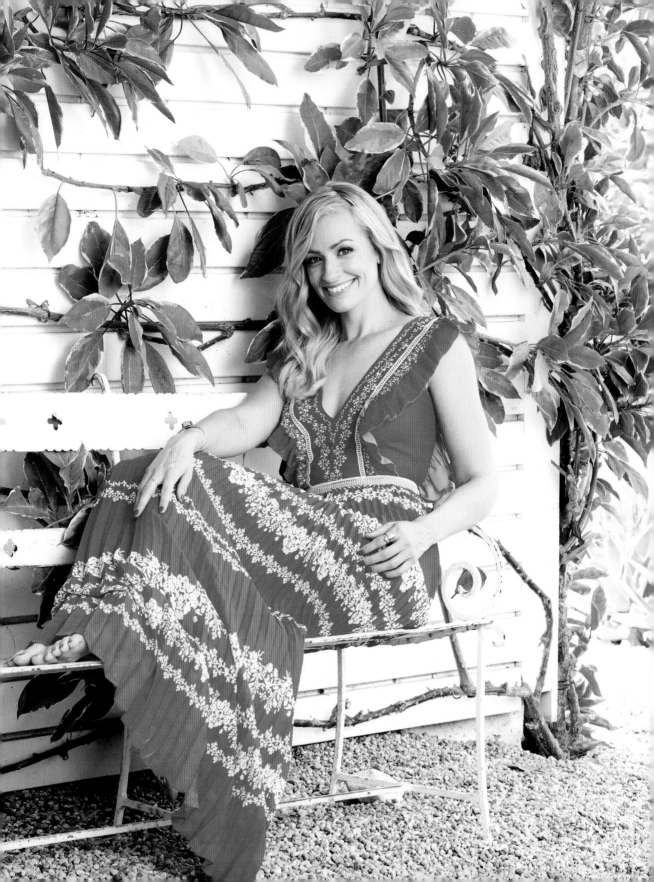

Part I

DITCH YOUR DIET

EVOLVING FROM JUNK-FOOD EATER TO JOYOUS FOODIE

I ate like a five-year-old boy until I was in my late twenties. Honestly. I had a friend who worked in a pizza kitchen, and she remembers me coming into the restaurant and ordering white pasta with red sauce on the side. I literally said, "No chunks in it!" Chunks being tomatoes. That's not just picky, that's like, INSANE. It's tomato sauce; a tiny bit of actual tomato should be acceptable. While my eating didn't impress anyone, luckily my skill on the playing field did. I was an athlete growing up. I bent it like Beckham on the soccer field—sort of—so excess weight was never really an issue.

I also loved junk food. In college, my roommate and I would get two sugar doughnuts each to keep us company on our mile-long walk to the theater department. Yes, please, mac and cheese and ramen. No, thank you, vegetables! I had never tried any leafy greens except for a plain hunk of iceberg lettuce. I ate green beans out of a can for my daily serving of veggies. My BFF and ex-roommate Courtney reminded me that when she met me, I not only ate the green beans directly from the can . . . I downed them WITH THE NASTY CAN LIQUID—and checked it off my list at night as my "greens for the day." (Calm down, men. I know I'm a catch.) I had no money and even less of a palate.

The only thing that ever temporarily busted me out of my white-bread, junk-food hole was, of course, boys. If I met a guy who was a foodie, I would try to impress him by eating Brussels sprouts. (Note to self: There are plenty of other things that will impress boys a lot more than eating Brussels sprouts. Like eating Brussels sprouts . . . naked. Or having a brain and saving the world, Amal Clooney–style.) But otherwise, my diet was pretty much all processed, all the time.

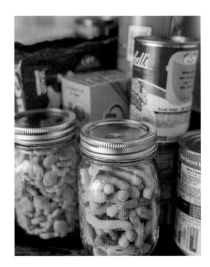

THE GROSSEST, MOST DELISH THINGS I USED TO EAT AND DRINK:

- TWO SUGAR-COVERED DOUGHNUTS (DAILY!) FROM THE UCLA COFFEE SHOP
- PIZZA!
- RAMEN
- CRONUTS (A LATECOMER, BUT OMG!)
- CHEESE (CHEDDAR, MUENSTER, GOUDA—YOU NAME IT.)
- PIZZA!
- FUNNEL CAKE (AT MY SCHOOL IN VIRGINIA—WHAT, YOUR SCHOOL DIDN'T HAVE FUNNEL CAKE?)
- CRÈPES WITH BUTTER, SUGAR, AND CINNAMON
- VELVEETA MAC AND CHEESE
- WHOLE BOXES OF SOUR PATCH STRAWS, DOTS, AND SNOW CAPS
- OK, PRETTY MUCH ANY CANDY
- OH, AND I FORGOT: PIZZA!

I reached my lowest point post-college. I ate and drank like I was on a reality show competition called *The Biggest, Drunkest Loser*. I was a couple of sizes bigger than I am now. That might not seem like such a big deal, but on my once-upon-a-time athletic and kind-of-short body, it was a very noticeable difference. Upside: My boobs looked great!

When I finally landed the gig on *2 Broke Girls*, I took to the craft service table—where they keep snacks and food on sets—like a long-lost friend. There were always candies, cookies, chips, and doughnuts for the scarfing . . . FOR FREE. During our first season of shooting, I noshed my way across that table daily. (Maybe that's why actresses are always on crazy diets—they're trying to compensate for the junk-food fest they have at work every day!) I was working crazy hours. My body was constantly sore from all the physical comedy I was doing on the show. I felt that "afternoon slump" as soon as I woke up. I stopped getting my period at the end of the first season. After being on set during the week, I was exhausted all weekend long, after memorizing up to sixty pages of script at a time. Finally, I went to a doctor, who ran some tests and discovered that I had a vitamin deficiency (shocker), along with an adrenal gland disorder from too much stress. (The adrenals, which rest on top of your kidneys, help you modulate stress by shooting out adrenaline, but they also help control your metabolism.) I wasn't living a healthy life, so I was unhealthy. Duh.

There was at least one really easy solution for this: Eat better, Beth. But human nature is funny. We *know* what's good for us. We *know* that when we eat well, exercise, and sleep well, we feel better. And yet—if someone puts a Dorito and a carrot in front of us, chances are we will eat the Dorito. What's wrong with us? Even though I knew better, I kept choosing the Dorito.

When I look back, I realize that it wasn't really about food; it was about what was happening in the moment. I was still new on the job and learning how to do it right. If I was performing in a scene and I didn't get the laugh because I didn't know the joke well enough to step on it and land it, then I walked out of the run-through feeling shitty. Baby carrots did not make me happy. But a Dorito gave me a quick hit of the Feel Goods. An instant fix—but a big mistake. So while I told the doctor I'd do my best, that still seemed to include very little exercise outside work and very many salty snacks.

A few months later, I got this weird rash. It started under my butt and migrated to my legs, a lovely place to have a rash! It looked like hives, but bigger and scalier and weirder—like Greyscale, *Game of Thrones*–style. I went to dermatologist after dermatologist, and they tried all sorts of things to get rid of it. At first they thought it was eczema, so they advised me to moisturize. So then I was moist (hate hate hate that word) *and* scaly. Then they tested me for psoriasis, and that was a dead end. A biopsy came back saying that it was a virus. Okay, we can treat a virus! I took a bunch of antibiotics, along with steroids, to try to bring down the inflammation. Four months later, it was spreading all over my back and the tops of my arms. On the show I wear this heinous miniskirt waitress uniform, and we had to cover my skin with body makeup. I had to cover my legs when I walked the red carpet (apologies to all those out there who lost an opportunity to ogle my gams). But what was most frustrating was that no meds worked. It was like having a cold that never went away . . . and makes you ugly from the neck down. Finally, my makeup artist recommended her specialist to me. She'd had terrible stomach problems and had gone to a doctor specializing in Auriculotherapy, an alternative Asian medical discipline that is like acupuncture in the ear. The doc also changed her diet, and she had amazing results. I thought if it worked for her, maybe it could work for me.

The practitioner used a special electrical tool to stimulate reflex points in my ear. He agreed that the rash was a virus, but as opposed to being caused by bacteria, he determined it was caused by deep stress. "Your immune system is shot," he told me and gave me a new and very limited diet plan. His instructions: "You are not allowed to have sugar, gluten, or dairy. Only lean protein, and I want you to pound spinach." (Maybe he didn't say "pound," but that's what he meant.) He also gave me a load of Chinese herbs. Doritos weren't on his list.

It wasn't easy, but I followed his directions to the letter. Within four days, the rash started disappearing from my legs. Holy wake-up call, Batman! I realized that I could never let my immune system get that weak again. If I let my body get stressed and my adrenals go to hell, then I couldn't do my work well, and I couldn't look and feel my best.

So I listened to that doctor. I followed his diet plan. The longer I stayed on my plan, the better I felt. It might sound like I conquered the impossible, but every time I lapsed—eating junk food or letting stress get the best of me—the skin virus came back.

It's tough to be that rigid and go cold turkey on the snacks we love and that give us comfort. While I could swing it for a few days, I had to do a fair share of experimentation and modification to find a long-term solution that felt right for me. For example, I had to include some additional animal proteins in my meals (which we'll talk about more later in this section). I also really, really paid attention to how my body felt after I ate. What digested easily? What tasted good? What left me feeling satisfied?

I didn't want to set any hard-core rules for myself because I wasn't interested in being on a diet. And once you make a rule—it's pretty easy to break. But with guidance from my doctor, a little online and anecdotal research, and some experimentation on my part, I came up with some guidelines for what to put in my body. I didn't make all these changes all at once, but slowly and surely I figured out a system that's been working for me:

- **Cut back on sugar/artificial sweeteners.** Sugar tastes great, but—it doesn't do much good for the body. In fact, it's pretty detrimental: It has no nutrients. It gets stored in your liver, where it turns into potentially harmful fat deposits, and it can raise the sugar levels in your blood to problematic levels. It hikes up the amount of insulin in your system, which taxes your arteries. It creates an energy surge in your system, followed by a crash. And then there's the damage it does to your skin and teeth . . . okay, fine, TOO MUCH SUGAR IS THE DEVIL. But you know what? I like that devil. So my thinking was: I'm not completely eradicating sugar from my diet, but I'll try to cut back and be more aware of added sugars in my food. I also stopped sprinkling little blue, pink, and yellow packets of artificial who-knows-what into my drinks. If I want something to taste sweeter, I use natural enhancers like honey or agave.
- **Scale back on diet soda.** I used to drink so, so much. But there are so many horrible chemicals in diet soda, which probably doesn't come as a surprise. (You totally read *Skinny Bitch*; I know you did!) So I kept some fizzy options (see page 53), but cut out diet soda.
- **(Don't) blame it on the alcohol.** I'll be honest with you—because all my friends know it—I'm a HUGE wino. Especially since I learned a little something about wine and upgraded from the boxed stuff to the good vino in bottles. I'm also nerdily into mixology and craft cocktails. But like all the other choices I make that affect my body, I try to curb my obsession and rein it in a little. The upside of a drink or cocktail can be the delicious taste and the fun, fizzy feeling that comes with it. The downside is that too many drinks lead to impaired judgment, especially when it comes to what edibles you're putting in your body. (Your good intentions to eat a light vegan lunch can quickly turn into a cheese-and-bread fest once you're feeling no pain.) Also, wine and all those super-fun cocktails can be a surprising source of sugar and excess calories—for example, a twelve-ounce frozen margarita can add up to

675 calories and eighty-three grams of sugar! Hard-core health experts (like the folks at the CDC) will tell you to limit your alcohol intake to a drink a day or less, or you can follow your own instincts and do your best to drink in . . . here it comes . . . moderation. (French people, I now give you permission to go ahead and laugh at me.) In my book (since this is my book), that means I raise a glass or two when the time is right—and stick to a drink here and there when full-on boozy celebration is not in order.

- **Have less "dairy" dairy and more "nondairy" dairy.** A lot of people are sensitive to dairy without being full-on lactose intolerant. It can cause bloating, digestion issues, fatigue, and allergy-like symptoms. For me, it exacerbates my sinus trouble. Plus, I realized that dairy was a source of added sugar in my diet. And once I realized that I could get calcium from leafy vegetables and legumes, and vitamin D from sunshine, I started to look for other "dairy-taste" sources, like nut milks and Greek yogurt (some Greek yogurt is made from goat's milk instead of cow's milk—check the label!—which is easier to digest). I still have a scoop of ice cream every now and then, but now I'm used to other options and I enjoy them.

- **Be aware of that gluten thing.** Just like dairy, you don't need to have full-on Celiac disease to be sensitive to gluten, a protein found in wheat, rye, and barley. For me, eating gluten can cause problems like lethargy and bloating. I feel better when I'm not eating bread and drinking beer, but again, I go with moderation.

- **Avoid processed foods.** I love me some chips and snacks; my body really doesn't. Our digestive systems weren't really designed to handle a lot of processed food, so I found that when I started to eat more whole and raw foods, I felt better. I had more energy. My stomach didn't feel unsettled. My skin and eyes appeared to look lighter and brighter. The truth is, you get barely any nutrition from a food made with stripped-down white flour or rice, or one that's made with simple sugars. Experts advise that you choose carbs that are full of fiber and digest slowly, to avoid spikes in blood sugar—think whole grains, veggies, fruits, and beans—so I use that rule of thumb. Brown rice is one of my favorite go-tos, as is quinoa pasta (throw a couple of garlic cloves into the quinoa pasta while you're boiling it for extra flavor).

- **Stop sprinkling salt.** Salt raises your blood pressure. So while I was already in the midst of getting rid of super-salty processed foods like chips and canned soups, I stopped giving that extra shake of the saltshaker over potatoes and other sides. I really don't miss it one bit because I season my food with all kinds of yummy things like herbs and spices.

- **Find alternatives to fat.** I was never the craziest fried-food fan, but I also didn't push away french fries when they showed up at the table. I still don't—but I don't go overboard. I generally try to stay away from saturated fats found in foods fried in oil. That means even my beloved doughnuts have become a rare treat. It wasn't a weight thing; it's that eating a lot of saturated fats puts you at a higher risk for heart disease. And now that I'm into "healthy" fats like olive oil, avocado, and nuts, I don't feel deprived when I decide to pass on my fried friends.

- **A little lean protein goes a long way.** I know plenty of people who feel great being on strictly vegetarian and vegan diets, but when I tried it, I found that I didn't have enough energy. So I try my best to eat a MOSTLY vegetarian diet. But I still have days when I feel like I need a small amount of animal protein to get the fuel I need. You'll find a lot of vegetarian and vegan recipes in these pages because there are some remarkable studies about how plant-based eating can ward off things like cardiovascular disease, diabetes, and cancer. But eating small amounts of well-sourced meat in moderation can have benefits, too. Nutritionist Maya Feller, MS, RD, CDN, CLC—a New York City–based registered dietitian nutritionist and owner of Maya Feller Nutrition Inc.—recommends eating a mix of wild-caught seafood, poultry, and lean meats. Make sure you're buying meat that is raised ethically, antibiotic- and hormone-free, and fed delicious pasture grass. How do you know? Ask your local butcher. Find someone you trust who can tell you all about their animal products, the farms they came from, and how they were raised. I have a butcher like that in my neighborhood, and we've discovered that we both value the humane treatment of animals.

LET'S GET COOKING

The biggest change wasn't what I ate, but how I ate it: I learned to cook. OMG, did I just say I *cooked*? I did! I am cool! I cook! I swear, I never thought cooking was something that I could do, but little by little I figured it out and I'll show you how it's done. Who knew that a day would come when I would have a better time shopping at Whole Foods than at Fred Segal? But it's true. I love going grocery shopping and learning to cook, and I swear, I *never* thought I'd say that. It's become a form of meditation for me—honestly! I relish time in the kitchen, whether it's by myself, with friends, or with my fiancé. I enjoy the process of taking a recipe I love and playing with it until it's just right for me. I look forward to putting on a record (favorites include Emmylou Harris and Johnny Cash, Stevie Wonder, Ella Fitzgerald sings Cole Porter, Al Green, The Rolling Stones, and The Beatles), drinking a glass of not-too-pricey Italian red, and cooking away. This is a huge step for me, because back in the day—okay, so like three years ago—I basically could burn water. Now I can't wait to share what I'm learning, and I'm seeing the difference that it can make in people's lives. When I sit down to eat that food that I've thought about and prepared, I always remember to take a minute and offer some gratitude for being able to eat what's good for me.

As my relationship with nutrition and health evolved, I realized that being healthy doesn't have to be all celery and suffering. I can enjoy what I eat, enjoy the lifestyle, and get my friends into it, too. Eating better doesn't just improve my energy, my mood, and my REGULARITY (that might be the best part), it also lowers my stress and makes me feel fulfilled. And all the stuff around it— shopping for produce, knowing my cumin from my curry, making a meal and sitting down to enjoy it—that's all part of being a grown-up. Part of getting my shit together. Part of living cleanly, me-toxing my body. Bidding good-bye to the kid who ate instant mac and cheese and embracing the adult who takes the time to feed herself the right way. Don't worry, I'm still a major dork. But I'm a dork who really values and respects myself and my body. That's a good thing.

This might be a good moment for you to think about the changes that you'd like to make in your own diet. I don't mean "diet" like the evil D-word that it is, but as the food that you eat on a daily basis. Are you looking to improve your overall level of nutrition by avoiding processed foods and excess sugar that can challenge your organs and leave you feeling achy, lethargic, and sick? Would you like to feel more strength and energy on a daily basis? Are you hoping to address physical challenges, everything from allergies to food sensitivities to skin problems? Would you like to eat healthier as a way to help our planet?

There are all sorts of ways to address the problems mentioned here, and this book will give you a few ways to start. Making changes *little by little* is the bottom line to all of this. It's hard to go full GOOP. But you CAN do little stuff here and there that builds up—like, for example, making your own salad dressing with ingredients already in your kitchen (see page 85). Start step by step and work your way up to good health. I promise that it will make a big difference in the long run. I've got clear skin and a happy mind to prove it!

HERE'S HOW YOU START: BIT BY BIT

Starting small really does mean starting small . . . and making changes so gradually that you hardly notice that you're actually making really big changes in the long run. I'll break this down into much more detail in chapter 1, but here's an example of three weeks of minor tweaks that can make a major difference:

DAY ONE: **Skip chips.** A day without salty snacks like chips, pretzels, and crackers. You can do that!

DAY TWO: **Skip sugar.** Go a day without *adding* sugar to anything you eat—and maybe make this a treat-free day. You can go for twenty-four hours without a cookie, piece of candy, or scoop of ice cream, right?

DAYS THREE–SEVEN: **Continue alternating as you did the first two days.** A day without salty snacks and then a day without sugar. If you find you can go without both for a day, do it!

DAY SEVEN: **Count up how much sugar you eat in a day.** While you're skipping the chips, tally up all the sugary treats you normally eat in a day. I'm not just talking about the spoonful of sugar you add to your coffee, but the amount of sugar you find in *all* the food you eat—including things like salad dressings, packaged sauces and soups, and bread. Yes, bread. Write down everything you eat today, then go online and add up the grams of sugar. Now, the American Heart Association (AHA) suggests that most women shouldn't eat more than twenty-four grams of added sugar per day (about six teaspoons). But the average American woman eats about *eighteen teaspoons* of added sugar a day. Nutritionist Maya Feller notes some frequent culprits, like heavily processed foods that are canned, frozen, jarred, or boxed. She also advises clients to look out for added sugar in cereals, granola bars, tomato and other sauces, yogurts, and condiments.

So try to find some places where you can cut the sugar out. For example, look at the label on the back of your morning yogurt: Holy hell, there are forty-three grams in that eight-ounce container? Dude, a Twinkie has only eighteen grams of sugar. Next time you're in the grocery store, try to find a yogurt that has less than eighteen grams of sugar in it and buy that one instead.

DAYS EIGHT–THIRTEEN: **Keep cutting down on that sugar** until you can get below that twenty-four-gram, or six-teaspoon, mark. And by this point, chips and salty snacks should be a rarity—maybe something you've grabbed one time in the week if you felt like you absolutely couldn't go without it.

DAYS FOURTEEN–SEVENTEEN: **Trade out white flour.** Go for something more fiber heavy, like whole wheat flour. That means wheat bread instead of white bread. Brown rice pasta instead of white pasta. And if you're a Rice Krispies eater, try a fiber-filled cereal instead.

DAYS EIGHTEEN–TWENTY-ONE: **Add in some greens**—fresh ones, not a can of GREEN BEANS IN NASTY LIQUID like, um, some people. Start with dark lettuce or iron-rich spinach—something easy to swap in for iceberg or throw on sandwiches. PS: The veggies in the freezer department of your grocery store have plenty of nutritional value and are easy to heat up if you're too time-crunched to cook. Try broccoli, Brussels sprouts, or sugar snap peas.

Suddenly, it's three weeks later and look at all the wonderful changes you've made! Your body is going to be like, "HELL YES—YOU DID IT!"

True, but chill out. You're not done yet. But the important thing is that you started, and all these small changes are about to add up to something big.

A NOTE ABOUT WEIGHT LOSS AND "DIETS"

I want to make it clear that this is not a weight-loss or diet book. You may find that when you clean out extra sugar and processed food from your intake, you lose weight, but that's not my intention here. I don't diet. I don't believe in diets. I do, however, believe that making moderate changes to the way you eat can lead to significant changes in the way you feel, and that's the guidance I'm trying to give you.

I also don't stick to any one particular "regime"—raw, vegan, Paleo, etc.—and would never recommend that you do either. It's all about what makes you feel good. I'll share all the wisdom that I've learned so far, but remember: Every body is different; you have to do what is right for yours.

I also highly recommend that anyone with a medical ailment should consult a doctor or nutritionist to see what kind of dietary changes are safe and beneficial.

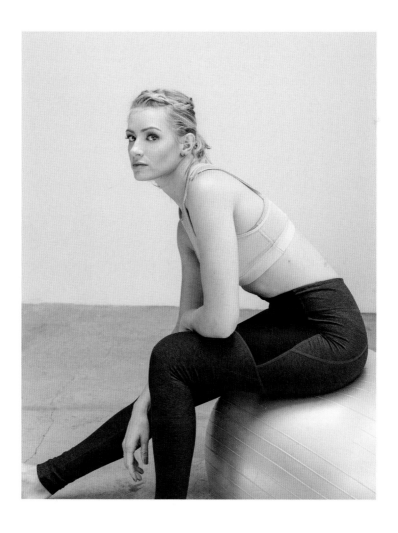

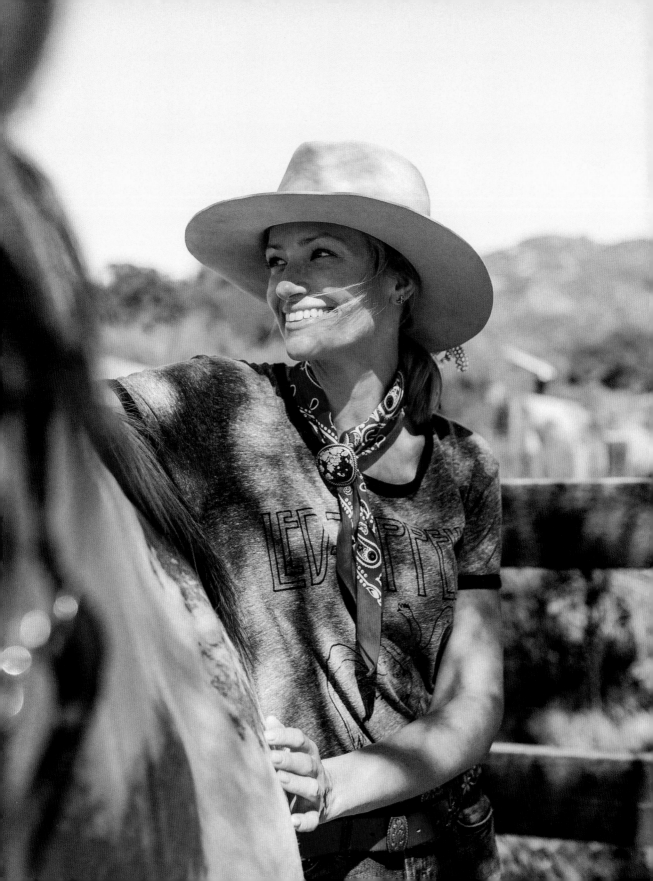

CHAPTER 1

STARTING SMALL

I often feel overwhelmed by a task because I always want to be the best at every-thing I do, and I want the end result RIGHT AWAY. For example, I've strug-gled with learning to play the guitar because I get frustrated and quit after two weeks when I find I can't strum, do the chord changes, and sing at the same time. But if I set smaller goals, say, two weeks just to work on the chords, the next two weeks to focus on strumming, and then add the singing, well, it makes my goal a lot more achievable. And it builds my confidence because I know the hard work is paying off. Bring on the Led Zeppelin! Bring on the classical Spanish guitar! Wait a second, Beth . . .

I'll give you the same advice when it comes to your health: Start small to make big goals come true. I've tried to address my health challenges week by week, kind of like playing that guitar. First you strum, then you work on the chords, then you amp up your Jimi Hendrix power ballads.

TIPS FOR STARTING SMALL

Set little, specific goals. Back this thang up a bit and ask yourself: What is my goal? For me, I had to get rid of a rash. But to get rid of the rash, I had to stop eating crap. And to stop wanting so much crap, I had to lower my stress. So bye stress, bye crap, bye rash. What are you trying to achieve? Clearer skin? Better nutrition? Better digestion? Getting food sensitivities in check? Healthier liv-ing in general? Stop for a second and give yourself a goal. If it's a major one ("I want to lose thirty pounds before my wedding," which PS, you don't have to do), then break it into smaller, more easily achievable pieces that will help you avoid frustration. How about, "I want to go one day without dairy products to see how I feel"? A weekend without beer? I'm talking *that* small.

Do your research. It can be a Google search or a coffee klatch with your friends, but get a little bit of info before you start making changes. If you're thinking about cutting excess sugar out of your diet, look up "What does sugar do to my body" to get a real sense of the physiology behind these changes. If you think you might want to eat less meat, ask a knowledgeable pal about "vegetarian versus vegan" to figure out which game plan would be the right one for you.

Schedule time . . . to shop. To cook. To eat. To clean up. You're never going to be able to jam a significant lifestyle change into the twenty minutes between leaving your office and getting to cocktails with the girls. Especially at the beginning, you need to make time to put your plan into action. So put it on your calendar and stick to it. I pick three nights a week when I know I am going to cook a meal. That also allows me to have leftovers of that healthy meal for lunch the next day. When it's in my schedule, it's less likely that I will get lazy and decide not to do it. (I've been doing the same thing with my workouts, which we'll get to later.)

For example, I go produce shopping on Sundays. (See produce-shopping tips on page 27.) We shoot on Mondays and Tuesdays. I used to order breakfast and lunch five days a week at work, but the novelty of ordering in wore off—and the calorie count was taking a toll. So now on Mondays and Tuesdays I usually bring something I've made at home, along with a carb. On Wednesdays I often go out to eat because, with my work schedule, Wednesday is my version of a Saturday. On Thursdays I generally bring breakfast and a lunch that includes a protein with brown rice, or a salad and veggies of some sort. On Fridays I try to eat healthy all day so I can indulge in a yummy dinner with friends on Friday evening. (BTW, Kat and I eat carbs. We have to. We once had these Victoria's Secret models on the show, with the craziest-looking bodies I have ever seen in my life. I took one look at them and said, "Yeah, I am *not* going to eat carbs." But literally halfway through the day I was like, "SOMEONE GO TO CHIPOTLE NOW AND GET ME RICE!" I realized that in order to run around in every scene, I needed carbs for energy.)

Add one healthy food habit each week. It can be increasing the amount of water you drink. Or putting sauce on the side of your veggies instead of pouring it over. You could try a morning ritual to start your day right—mine includes drinking hot water with lemon before I put anything else in my body. I find that when I start my day off right, it continues right. And by making it a habit, every day gets off on the right foot.

Embrace your bitchin' kitchen. Your kitchen is more than a storage spot for a refrigerator that only has mustard, beer, and old Chinese takeout in it. The major thing that people do in the kitchen is cook. That's right, cook. I know most people in our generation spend more time watching cooking shows than doing actual cooking—I was one of them. For so many reasons I'd talked myself out of thinking that I had the time, energy, or skill to cook. But like all the suggestions above, I started small by making smoothies and snacks and built my way up to sides and meals. It was the key to improving my health and changing my life. And you can do it, too.

> *Beth, it sounds really rational and sensible and doable when you explain it like this.*
> Good!
> *And you seem like a lovely person.*
> Awww, thanks.
> *But there's no way I can do what you did.*
> Oh, really? Try me . . .
> *I can maybe get some good food habits going, but I've got a whole list of reasons why I can't cook.*
> Oh, really? How about this: You give me the excuse . . .
> *I said "reason."*
> No, it's an excuse.
> *Okay.*
> So you give me the excuse, and I'll prove to you that it can be done.
> *Umm . . .*
> Ready? Go.

I CAN'T COOK 'CAUSE . . .

I really don't want to.
Been there, done that. But if you try it once, then you might find that you actually like it. You can do stuff you like while you cook—like talk on the phone, watch Bravo, or listen to music. We will make this nice for you.

I'm so incredibly tired.
I feel you. The craziest thing is that making a nice, healthy meal for yourself is going to give you *more* energy.

I'm a feminist.
I am, too. You can be a feminist and still cook. No one is forcing you to "stay in the kitchen." You are making a positive choice for yourself and your future, and if that's not a feminist act, nothing is.

It's too hot to turn on the oven.
Oh, it definitely is! Especially if you're cooking in a tiny little apartment. But there are things that you can make that do not require an oven, or even heat (see page 37). And soon you'll be such a pro at whipping up quick meals that you can get the oven involved, no sweat.

I don't know what to make.
I have lots of ideas for you in this book! Check out page 108 for tons of my favorite recipes.

I didn't go to the grocery store.
I'm sure there's stuff we can find in your house (see page 24).

I have nothing in the house.
Hmm, really. Nothing? Like, capture-a-mouse-for-dinner nothing? That's why they invented Instacart, Amazon Fresh, and Postmates!

Well, nothing I have in the house appeals to me.

Sure, I get that. How 'bout we decide that this particular meal doesn't have to be the be-all, end-all in the great-taste department and just put some healthy fuel in your body and try again tomorrow?

I don't know how.

I'm going to show you! You don't even have to start with a whole meal—it could be a simple snack instead.

I don't have time.

You're right. Nobody has time. That's part of the reason we're all so sick and tired and stressed out. So we're going to make a little time. You don't have to make a lifetime commitment, but can you pick ONE HOUR this week to dedicate to doing something really, really kind for yourself and your body? You have 168 hours this week. Can we give ONE of them to you? It's going to be worth it.

I'm telling you, it ain't happening tonight.

Okay, how about finding a restaurant that serves food you won't feel bad about eating? There's this healthy Indian place near me that I order from when a home-cooked meal just isn't in the cards. It's not perfect, but I don't have to feel bad about it either.

I'm eating alone—cooking is a waste of food.

None of the recipes in this book will go to waste. Tonight's dinner is tomorrow's lunch. Or next week's dinner if you freeze leftovers. Or a nice offering to a neighbor.

People make fun of my cooking.

F 'em.

I can't afford to buy a lot of ingredients.

Believe me, I was there. I've included a lot of ideas for good, cheap meals in this book. And get this—cooking, especially from whole ingredients, is way less expensive than ordering takeout or buying a lot of packaged products.

I'm scared. I don't even know how to start.
Yeah, you do. You're going to start small.

See, there's really no excuse. But if you're really stressing about getting comfortable in the kitchen, do what I did and make the change in three basic steps:

1. **Start simple** with stuff like smoothies, drinks, and snacks.
2. **Maximize meals** by starting to cook your own easy, super-healthy dishes.
3. **Invite others** to join you in the process.

Now, it's going to be tough for you to wake up tomorrow morning and start from scratch. So before you start smoothie-ing and snacking, you need to get set up. In the next chapter I'll give you the lowdown on everything you'll need to get prepped, from gearing up your kitchen to shopping for food.

By the way, you don't have to wait until tomorrow morning to shift gears. It could be even tougher to turn yourself around if you have one of those "I'm going to consume all the candy/cake/fried chicken/beer I can get my hands on" last-blast meals tonight, so don't go crazy, 'kay? Remember: Your goal is to slowly but surely make micro-changes that lead to macro living. I believe that doing a little something beneficial for yourself trumps doing nothing at all. So fine, you had a tube of Pringles. Instead of being like, "THERE GOES THAT DAY," make yourself a little chicken and spinach for dinner! (This is what my friends call a "Whoa, Girl" moment, as in "Whooooooa, don't be so hard on yourself, girl!" Sometimes you gotta step back, give yourself credit for the thing you did right, and let the bad moment float away like a little bubble in the sky.) It didn't happen overnight for me. It took me three and a half years to get where I am now. And even now, I stumble and feel my way through. Like, I recently went to the movies and decided that it would be a super-delicious idea to eat a box of Sour Patch Kids. How *good* are Sour Patch Kids? So good! But I have been off sugar for a long-ass time, and they made me SO SICK. Halfway through *Star Wars: The Force Awakens* I felt like I had chunks of BB-8 rolling around in my stomach. I was nauseous, and my head was pounding. But I'm not going to go all Kylo Ren and beat myself up about it. (Whoa, girl!) Next time I want a movie treat, I'll order popcorn, no butter. No drama—it just wasn't a good idea for my body, and I know that now. But I have plenty of good ideas for your body that have really worked for me, and they start now.

CHAPTER 2

GETTING STARTED (A.K.A. KITCHEN *SECRETS OF THE ANTI-MARTHA*)

You know those movies where someone starts a new job—a teacher or the assistant to the dazzling-yet-intimidating Prada-wearing Devil—and the first scene is them setting up their workplace? Sitting down in the chair, giving it a spin, putting out their nameplate or boxed lunch? That's you! Setting up your workspace—your kitchen—is a great first step when you're going to make changes in your life, especially when it comes to eating. You're going to find it's helpful to be really deliberate about what you're doing and to plan in advance what you're going to eat and when you're going to eat it. It's not about being rigid; it's about being *prepared*. This way, when you're super hungry, you'll have healthy snacks or a wholesome meal on hand, which will make it more difficult to cave and run to the nearest fast-food place. Or when you get home from work or school and you're too pooped to start prepping a meal, you'll already have produce cut up and ready to go. When you've made changes in your kitchen, your brain will follow.

It's bizarre to even hear myself talking this way. When my fiancé Michael and I first met, I didn't know the first thing about the kitchen. At the time, I was super poor and—as I've previously confessed—I tended to eat food that would appeal to anybody watching the Disney Channel. My cooking and eating repertoire included mac and cheese and hot dogs—and that about covers it. Michael, on the other hand, had great taste and a good income. One night he took me to an incredible restaurant where they served these roasted peppers . . . oh, those peppers, crispy and hot and sweet . . . I was instantly obsessed. To my surprise,

Michael said they were easy to make. "You buy a few peppers, wash them, put them in some hot oil in a pan, add a little bit of salt and pepper, and cook them until they shrivel." So later I went to the store and got some peppers that looked like what I'd had at the restaurant. I was pushing my limits. Trying something new. Impressing the guy. More important, impressing myself. And I felt cool. I went home, washed 'em up, put them in the pan with the oil, salt, and pepper. They shriveled and looked just like the ones we had eaten at the restaurant! I was thinking, *This isn't so hard! Next up, standing rib roast.* I started to eat them, maybe three or four. Mmm, good. Good and hot. Whoa, very hot. HOLY $#*! THESE ARE CRAZY HOT!

What I had bought were serrano peppers, about five times hotter than jalapeños, which are about five times hotter than shishitos—the kind they were serving at the restaurant. I stayed up sick all night while Michael held my hair back and praised me for at least trying something new. (Maybe that was the beautiful moment when he really fell for me.)

But again, life lessons show up in weird ways. I learned that I couldn't get ahead of myself. Maybe I needed to start by boiling water instead of pan-frying peppers. So I advise you to do the same: Start slow, take your time, build up. Prepare your space. Up your cooking game on your own schedule.

If I can do it, anybody can. I've learned how to eat super healthfully, creatively, and deliciously. But in order to get here, I had to get prepared. Get geared up. Go grocery shopping. This chapter is your guide for doing just that.

GEARING UP

Back in the day, when you became a young married lady, you had a wedding shower and everyone supplied you with all the necessities for a long and successful career in homemaking. Well, those days are over. While you might still have a wedding shower at some point, you'll likely collect your own pots, pans, and dishes over time. The pots, pans, and dishes that I'm bringing into married life are super gnarly.

I have to admit that I get a lot of pleasure from having matching silverware and a full set of functional measuring cups. All that aesthetically pleasing stuff is another motivator to get me going in the kitchen. But it's in no way essential to learning how to cook, or to enjoying the process. However, if you're looking to start gathering some good kitchen gear, or fill in some blanks, here's a handy checklist. Don't feel like you need to spend a million bucks or have the most high-end gear on the market. You can find great deals online. You can buy items at garage sales. You can ask your mom or grandma to part with the stuff they got for their showers and never use. Or, the next time you have a birthday, graduation, or Chrismukkah, create a "registry" and have your friends give you something you know you'll put to good use. You don't need to put a ring on it to get your kitchen fired up.

In the Drawer
- Aluminum foil
- Plastic wrap
- Resealable plastic bags (assorted sizes)
- Dish towels (instead of paper towels)
- The Honest Company or Mrs. Meyer's dish soap (no nasty chemicals!)
- Utility scissors or kitchen shears

For Baking and Cooking
- Casserole dish with lid
- Big, deep skillet
- Smaller nonstick frying pan
- Big-ass pot with lid
- Medium pot with lid
- Small/sauce pot with lid
  Note: You can often find a stainless-steel or nonstick porcelain or enamel cookware set that includes all of the above!
- Nonstick baking sheets (two)
- Glass bakeware set that includes baking dishes
- Cupcake tins
- Loaf pan
- Colander
- Cutting boards: one for meat and one for everything else (I like plastic for meat and wood for veggies, cheese, fruit, etc.)

- Vitamix, NutriBullet, or other blender
- Set of mixing bowls (I prefer a couple of nice, durable stainless-steel ones for when I use my KitchenAid mixer—the KitchenAid is not essential, but very useful.)
- Pot holders/oven mitts (Silicone is great, but I prefer quilted because my aunt Meme [the nun—see the story on page 148] sewed her own as presents for us. Cooking with love!)
- Mason jars: four 8-ounce jars and two 16-ounce jars (For smoothies, chlorophyll water, coconut water, storing spices and dry goods, you name it. You can buy them cheaply in bulk on Amazon. They look super chic and hipster on the shelf/counter.)

Utensils

- Knives: chef, paring, and serrated
- Sharpening stone (Sharp knives are not only helpful—they chop veggie-cutting time in half—but also important. One night when Michael was out of town, I made the brilliant move of trying to pull a pit out of an avocado by sticking the point of my knife into it. I ended up slicing open my finger instead. At the ER the doctor said admiringly, "It's a beautiful cut . . . you must have really sharp knives!" He assured me that the cut would heal quickly due to his ability to stitch up that smooth line. Michael takes a weird kind of pride in this story. On dates when we'd be cooking together, he'd come over WITH HIS OWN SHARPENING STONE. He bought his mom one as a gift, too. The moral of the story? Show your love with very, very sharp instruments.)
- Whisk
- Tongs
- Rubber or silicone spatula
- Vegetable peeler
- Corkscrew
- Can opener
- Ladle
- Slotted spoon
- Wooden spoon—use it for EVERYTHING

- Grater
- Set of measuring spoons
- Set of measuring cups (for dry measures)
- Two-cup Pyrex measuring cup (for liquid measures)
- Baby-bottle brushes (to clean those mason jars)
- Handheld lemon juicer (for morning-lemon-water convenience)
- Little wooden bowls (for black pepper, kosher salt, or other spices—I keep one right near the stove so it's easy to grab a quick pinch.)
- Sponges (I buy the scrub-top ones at the grocery store or get them in bulk at Costco. Wash 'em in the dishwasher if you're worried about germs, or just replace them frequently.)

START SHOPPING

Before you go all Giada, you should stock up on some basic items for your pantry that will help you make a lot of different meals, without a lot of effort. Here is a shopping list for staples:

Oils, Vinegars, and Condiments

- Oils: canola, extra-virgin olive, coconut
- Vinegars: balsamic, distilled white, red wine, rice, apple cider
- Dijon mustard
- Soy sauce (low-sodium)
- Chili paste
- Hot sauce
- Worcestershire sauce

Seasonings

- Black peppercorns
- Kosher salt
- Dried herbs, spices, and spice blends: bay leaves, cayenne pepper, red pepper flakes, ground cumin, ground coriander, oregano, paprika, rosemary, thyme, chili powder, curry powder, Italian seasoning, garlic powder, cinnamon, cloves, allspice, ginger, nutmeg (see Spice Up Your Life, page 34)

Canned Goods and Other Pantry Items

- Canned beans: black, cannellini, chickpeas, kidney
- Low-sodium stock or broth (I especially like bone broth.)
- Tomatoes, canned and paste
- Capers
- Olives
- Almond butter (If you're going to buy it, try Justin's all-natural version.)
- Brown rice cakes
- Dried fruit: raisins, mango, apricots
- Nuts and seeds: almonds, peanuts, sunflower

Grains and Legumes

- Couscous
- Brown rice
- Rolled oats
- Barley
- Millet
- Quinoa
- Wheat berries
- Dried lentils
- Whole wheat pasta

Baking Products
- Baking powder
- Baking soda
- Brown sugar
- Cornstarch
- Flour (wheat or almond)
- Honey
- Vanilla extract

Refrigerator Basics
- Large eggs (worth splurging on organic; good for about a month)
- FAGE Total 0% Greek yogurt (It doesn't have to be FAGE, but that's my favorite brand.)

Freezer Basics
- Frozen fruit: raspberries, blueberries, strawberries, mango, pineapple
- Frozen vegetables: broccoli, bell pepper and onion mix, edamame, peas, spinach

Storage Produce
- Garlic
- Onions (red and yellow)
- Potatoes (sweet and regular)
- Lemons
- Fresh ginger

WEEKLY SHOPPING TRIPS

Once you have your kitchen stocked with the basics, the only things left to buy are fresh provisions for about a week's worth of meals. After a few weeks in your new routine, you'll realize that your list of essentials looks similar from week to week, so shopping will get that much quicker and easier.

Here's a recent shopping list of mine that I used to buy about a week's worth of groceries:

1 box Erewhon unsalted,
   unbuttered organic popcorn

4 apples

1 pint blueberries

1 big bunch green grapes

1 bag baby carrot sticks
   (great for dipping in
   Yummy Hummus, page 67)

2 boxes organic baby spinach
   (for salads or as side vegetable)

1 bunch fresh kale

2 cucumbers
   (for salads or as snack)

5 ribs celery
   (for snacking or dipping)

1 bag sugar snap peas

3 onions

2 heads garlic

2 jalapeño peppers

3 red bell peppers
   (for dips, salads, or adding
   to Anything Goes Frittata,
   page 136)

4 chicken breasts
   (for No-Frills "Gourmet" Chicken,
   page 122)

½ pound lean ground turkey
   (for turkey burgers, turkey
   meatballs, or turkey chili)

PRODUCE SHOPPING 101

You might notice that your trips to the grocery store are changing—you're probably spending a lot more time in the fresh produce section than in the middle of the store, with all the processed food. While you're chilling near the lettuce heads, let me offer you some hints on how to shop for produce and how to store your goods once you get home so they last as long as possible. (It sucks to spend big $ on produce and just throw it out!)

General Tips

Buy in season. You'll notice that berries cost twice as much during the winter, because it costs that much more to ship them to you from California or Florida, where most of them are grown. And it's going to be hard to buy a pumpkin around Easter, since patches don't start going full-on Charlie Brown until the fall. Plus, stuff grown out of season just doesn't taste as good. So do yourself, your wallet, and your carbon footprint a favor and enjoy your produce when the season is right.

Buy what you'll eat. I know you're excited to jump into these new recipes, but don't go too crazy. Buy what you think you'll *really* consume. I'm all about getting ambitious, but keep in mind that most fresh veggies will only last around 2 to 5 days. That said, root vegetables like potatoes and squash can last a week or more. Apples, onions, and citrus have a decent shelf life, too.

Don't blanch at a bump. We've been conditioned to think that good produce has to look shiny and perfect, but then again, we've been conditioned to think that WE have to look shiny and perfect. Most produce has a tiny bit of wear and tear, and that's just fine . . . especially if it's been grown without the use of heavy pesticides.

Shop at a farmers' market. You'll not only be supporting local farmers who use fewer or no pesticides to keep produce healthy, but you'll also be able to ask them how fresh the produce is! IMHO, their stuff tastes better than grocery store produce.

Artichokes: Choose 'chokes that are small and feel a teeny bit heavy in your hand, with leaves that squeak a little when you squeeze them. California artichokes are usually available year-round, but peak season is March through May. Sprinkle them with a little bit of water and store in a plastic bag in your fridge—they should last for about a week.

Asparagus: Go for smooth-looking stalks with closed tips and bright green color; they're especially fresh in the spring. You can store asparagus spears in the fridge standing upright in a glass with an inch of water in it, like a little bouquet of flowers, and they'll last for a couple of days.

Avocado: If it feels squishy, that avocado is overripe. Pass! If it feels rock-hard, it's not ready to go. To help it ripen, leave it in a bowl with apples or bananas. (Fun fact: Apples and bananas emit gasses that cause the fruit around them to ripen more quickly.) Once they are ripe, store them in the fridge and they'll stay fresh for about a week. You can find avocados year-round.

Bananas: Buy them when they still have a tiny bit of a green hue; they'll keep ripening when you get them home. Remember to keep them away from other fruit if you want both them and the other fruit to last longer. When they start to turn brown, peel them and store them in a plastic bag in the freezer for smoothies.

Beets: They should be firm and have a bright red or orange color. White spots are a no-no. Beets are in season in spring and fall, and they'll stay fresh in your refrigerator for almost two weeks.

Broccoli: Look for heads that are firm and compact, with a bright or deep green color. Yellow is not a good sign. Don't yield for yellow. Broccoli is available year-round, but peak season is October to April. Keep it in a bag in your vegetable drawer, and it should stay good for up to ten days.

Brussels sprouts: You want bright green sprouts with tight leaves. The smaller the sprouts, the more tender they'll be. Peak season runs from September to mid-February, but you can generally find them year-round. Refrigerate them, and you'll get the best taste if you eat them within three to four days.

Cabbage: It should be firm and feel heavy in your hand. See Beth's Field Guide to Common Greens (page 87) for more info.

Cantaloupe: Give it a whiff—it should smell sweet, but not too sweet; too sweet means overripe, and you want to get as much mileage out of it as you can. If it feels really hard, you can let it ripen a bit more on your countertop. PS: Shake a cantaloupe next to your ear before you buy it. It won't make a damn difference, but you'll sure look like you know what you're doing. Summertime is cantaloupe time; it's tastiest from June through August.

Carrots: You might assume that you want the ones that look smooth and firm, with a nice orange color. You know, like a snack Bugs Bunny would want to gnaw on. But those knobby ones from the farmers' market are just as awesome. And if you haven't tasted yellow or purple carrots, get on that! You can find carrots at the market pretty much year-round, but fall is their optimal season. Store the greens separately because they can cause carrots to spoil more quickly (you can use them in soups and salads!), and keep the carrots in an open plastic bag in the fridge. They're a hardy veg and should stay good for up to two weeks.

Cauliflower: Go for white- or cream-colored tight curds (I've always wanted tighter curds) that have nice green jackets surrounding them. Cauliflower knows how to accessorize. It's available year-round, but peak season is the fall. Wash it as you eat it, and keep the rest in the refrigerator, stem-side up, for up to five days.

Celery: Pick firm stalks with a light- to medium-green color and a little bit of a glossy look. They're available all year, but mid- to-late summer is prime time. Stash in the fridge for up to a week and slice just before using.

Citrus (lemons, limes, oranges, grapefruits): You want bright color and smooth skin that feels a little springy to the touch. Note: You don't have to get the biggest one in the bin; sometimes big = watery. And by all means, give your citrus a sniff; it has such a nice scent! Any time is a good time to buy citrus, but late winter is primo. Lemons, limes, oranges, and grapefruits will stay fresh at room temperature for about a week, and you can extend their life in the fridge for another week.

Corn (in the husk): Look for tight green husks. The silk flowing out of the husks should be a light color and not too brown. Corn at the market means summertime is here! Store it in the refrigerator unshucked and eat it within two days of buying it for the sweetest flavor.

Cucumbers: Pick cukes with a vibrant green color that feel firm from top to bottom. Stroke that cucumber—it's not illegal. (By the way, I figured out only recently that a pickle was really a pickled cucumber. So you can see how badly I need this kind of information.) You'll find them year-round, but peak season is May through July. Store cucumbers at room temperature; they'll only stay fresh in the refrigerator for up to three days.

Eggplant: So good to cook with. You can pick the classic ones with a dark-purple jewel color or give white or speckled varieties a try. Ripe eggplants should feel firm and smooth. They're available year-round, but July to October is peak eggplant time. Keep them on the countertop (not in the refrigerator). They're good for up to three days.

Grapes: They should be firm and stay on the stem when you give them a tiny (tiny) tug. Yes, you can taste one at the store—but be sure to rinse them well when you bring them home! You can buy grapes year-round, but California grapes are only available from July to November. They'll stay fresh in the fridge for about a week, but only wash them as you use them.

Greens: You want them to look fresh, tender, and—it should go without saying—green, without any soggy brown bits. See Beth's Field Guide to Common Greens (page 87) for more info.

Green/string beans: Obvs not from a can. Select the smoothest, greenest ones out of the bin. They're in season all summer long, and they'll keep in your fridge for up to a week.

Leeks: These should be dark green and firm at the top and white at the bulb end, with crisp-looking "fringe" still attached. In season October through May (peaking in January), they'll last for up to a week in your fridge.

Lettuce: Whether you go loose or buy a head, buy bright, firm varieties that don't look wilted or brown. It's okay to buy lettuce in a bag, but bagged lettuce rarely lasts as long as its expiration date. See Beth's Field Guide to Common Greens (page 87) for more info.

Mangoes: They can be green or orangey-yellow, depending on what kind you like. The perfect day for mango-eating is when they feel firm with just a little give and smell delish. Wait for them to get super soft, and it'll be a day too late. If you want a mango to ripen more, keep it out on the counter. There are all different ways to cut a mango; just look online for demos. But remember to use a sharp knife! Mangoes have two seasons, spring/summer and fall/winter, so you should be able to find them all year.

Mushrooms: You can buy many different kinds, including white, shiitake, cremini, or portobello. Broken 'shrooms and mushy spots are no good. You can find mushrooms all year long, but fall/winter is generally the tastiest season. Store them unwashed in the fridge in a single layer under a damp paper towel for up to three days.

Okra: They should be a little bendy in your hand but not completely soft. Early fall is the ideal time for okra. Refrigerate them unwashed for two to three days or freeze for months.

Onions: Whether yellow, white, or red, onion skins should be shiny and tight. And remember when cutting them: sharp knife = fewer tears. Store them in a dry, cool place and they'll last you a while. You can buy them year-round, but they tend to be lighter in the spring/summer and denser in the fall/winter. Keep them in a cool, dry, ventilated spot (but not the fridge) for two to three weeks.

Peppers (bell): Go for brightly colored peppers (red, yellow, orange, and green) that are a little bigger than your hand. They should feel firm to the touch with a little bit of gloss to them. They're best in the late summer months but available year-round. Keep them unwashed in a plastic bag in your fridge's veggie drawer. Reds and yellows will last four to five days; greens can go about a week.

Potatoes: It's okay if potatoes have little spots here and there (like eyes), but they shouldn't have areas of "sunburn." Sweet potatoes and yams should have a uniform color. Don't buy them too big, or they could be more watery and less tasty. There are many varieties to choose from, but round red potatoes are great for boiling and roasting, and russets are ideal for baked and mashed recipes. You can find them year-round, but potatoes are best from late summer through the fall. Keep them in a dark, dry place (the refrigerator is too cold!), and they'll keep for several months. If you get little sprouts on them, cut them away before cooking and eating.

Radishes: Choose the ones that are about ¾ to one inch in diameter, with a plump look and a nice ruby color. Great for raw dipping. Radishes are available year-round but peak in springtime. Cut off the greens and store the roots (the red part) in the crisper drawer for up to a week.

Snow peas/sugar snap peas: These are fun to eat because you can eat both the shell and the little peas inside. They're in season during the spring and fall. If you refrigerate them in a baggie with a moist paper towel in it, they'll stay fresh for up to five days.

Squash: So many ways to squash! Remember that spaghetti squash is stringy (duh), butternut is creamy (a lot like sweet potatoes), buttercup is dry and crumbly, and acorn is dense and fibrous, which is ideal for soups, stews, and casseroles. Plus, squash looks cute on your countertop. Summer squashes are available in the summer and winter squashes in the . . . you guessed it, winter! They'll stay fresh in a dry, cool place for months.

Stone fruits (cherries, nectarines, peaches, and plums): They're called "stone fruits" for the pit in the middle. They should have nice, smooth, clear surfaces.

And if they're rock-hard, they're not ripe! May through September is their season, but the peak is July/August. Stone fruits will last for three to four days at room temperature and five to six in the fridge (if they're already ripe).

Strawberries: Usually the smaller the tastier! They should have a nice jewel red color and will smell really delicious when they're at perfect ripeness. Rinse them well just before eating—they only last for a day or two with the stems cut off. (Same for blueberries, blackberries, and raspberries—they'll last longer if you wait to wash them.) Strawberries are in season from late spring through the summer.

Tomatoes: When they're bright red, they're really ripe. Look for smooth, shiny skin. But don't be afraid to try some "interesting"-looking tomatoes at the farmers' market or to pop some cherry tomatoes in your shopping bag. Summertime is ideal tomato time, from June to September. There's some debate about whether you should store tomatoes in the refrigerator, but if they're ripe when you buy them, they'll be fine in the fridge for about four days. If you're not going to use them right away, tomatoes can still have a little pink tone to them and will continue to ripen a bit if kept on the counter or in sunlight (not in the fridge).

Watermelon: Give your melon a slap; it should have a slightly hollow sound when it's ripe. Special watermelon exception to the rule: It doesn't need to have a perfect skin to have a delicious taste—it gets rolled around a lot in transit from the watermelon patch to your place. Watermelon is available year-round but at its prime in August, which is why you might think of it as a summer fruit. Store your uncut melon in a cool, dry place for up to a week; once you cut it up, it will only stay crisp in the fridge for three to four days.

STUMP YOUR PALS

Which one's a parsnip and which one's a turnip?
   A parsnip looks like a white carrot and has the consistency of a carrot when you cook it. A turnip looks like a radish but cooks and tastes a little bit more like a potato.

SPICE UP YOUR LIFE: MOVING BEYOND SALT AND PEPPER

I'm a total spice girl. If I were in the Spice Girls, I'd be Spicy Spice. It's not just a matter of taste; the spice thing helps me to eat healthy because I need a ton of flavor. Plus, spices are super affordable and you can throw them in anything. Add a few Indian spices like cumin or freshly ground turmeric to your spinach, or sprinkle some chiles on cauliflower or string beans, then put them on a baking sheet with a little oil and roast them at 350°F for ten minutes; you get your veggies in, and they just taste so much better.

Here are some of my favorite herbs, spices, spice mixes, and aromatics and how I use them:

Bay leaves: Literally, add them to EVERYTHING for some extra flavor: spaghetti sauce, soups, sauces. I even add them to the water I use to cook veggies or pasta. Virgin bay leaf users take note: Remove the leaves from the pot or pan before serving the food—you're not supposed to ingest them.

Garam masala: You'll find this spice blend in my chicken (or lentil) saagwala recipe on page 111. It's aromatic, sweet, and warm—my favorite of all the Indian spices.

Garlic: Just call me Stinky Behrs, because I add garlic to everything I make . . . like, one or two cloves more than the recipe calls for. And I eat 'em whole when I'm getting sick (see page 172). Hey, want to make out? Pro tip: After you crush or chop garlic, let it sit for about fifteen minutes to really activate all the compounds that give your dish great flavor.

Ginger: Um, see GARLIC. As in, USE GINGER IN EVERYTHING. Add it to smoothies every morning or use it in tea as a cold fighter and to help digestion (it "heats up" your tummy).

Marash and aleppo pepper: These are two types of ground chile peppers that I found at my local spice shop. They are incredible in anything and everything. I use them for a spicy kick in almost every dish I cook. I wish I could stash them in my purse and add them to dishes when I go out to eat. Wait, that's not a bad idea . . .

Paprika: Add to your sweet potato fries, hummus, omelets—anything where you want some subtle spice. For a little smokiness, buy smoked paprika. It reminds me of being outdoors in the fall, my favorite time of year.

Rosemary: I grow it right outside my kitchen and use it as flavoring for chicken, pasta, and salad dressings as well as a pretty garnish for omelets. Some of its fresh, herby cousins include thyme, oregano, sage, dill, parsley, and tarragon.

Turmeric: A staple at my house. I sometimes add it to my smoothies, and I swear by Turmeric Tea (page 52). You can peel and chop the fresh root, or use the powder form, which is amazing for cooking curry dishes and other ethnic eats. Even though it doesn't have a ton of flavor on its own, it's an amazing anti-inflammatory/disease-fighting/anti-aging helper. Heads up: It will stain your cutting board, nails, fingers, et al. . . . but it's worth it! Just scrub it out with a little soap and water.

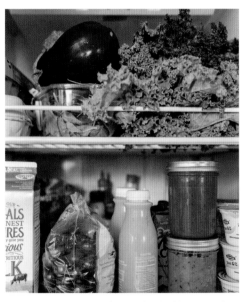

What Beth's pantry/fridge looks like now that she's maximizing meals.

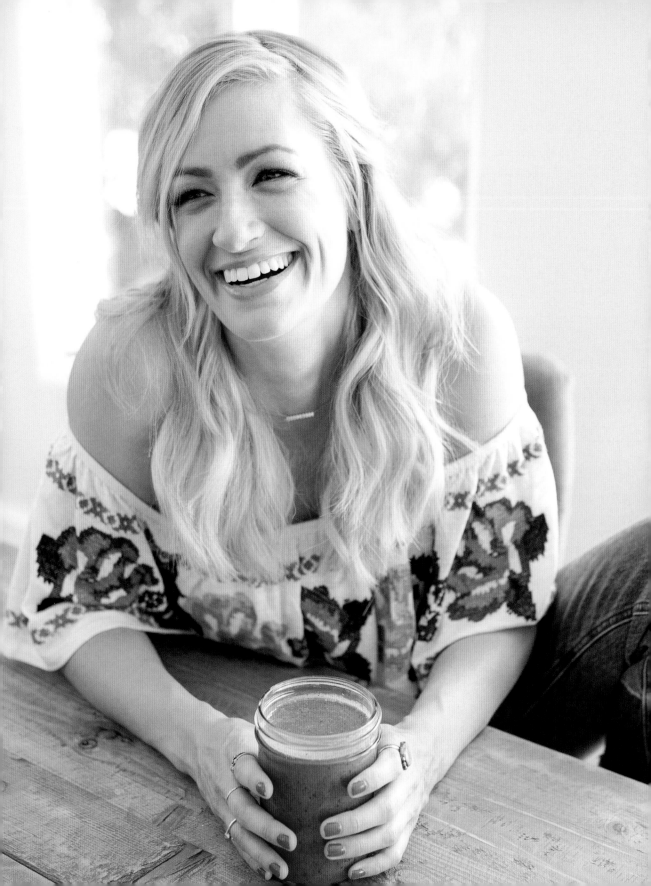

CHAPTER 3

START SIMPLE:
SMOOTHIES, DRINKS & SNACKS

I'm serious about starting small. You don't need to make a nine-course Thanksgiving feast your first day out—start instead with smoothies, drinks, and snacks! Smoothies in particular are like a gateway drug into cleaner eating, and they're so quick and easy to make. (And once I started smoothie-ing it, I noticed less cellulite. The greener and more nutrient-rich the veggies I ate, and the more raw or pure the food I was eating, the more my dimples shrunk!) Bumping up your intake of clean drinks like water and tea is going to increase your energy, reduce your risk of high blood pressure and high cholesterol, keep your skin bright, and improve your digestion by flushing out unwanted bacteria. And switching up your snacks—away from processed junk food and toward whole foods, fruits, and vegetables—will flood your body with nutrients and energy.

SMOOTHIE & DRINK RECIPES

I'd always heard that drinking smoothies was a good strategy for improving my health, but I never wanted to wake up early to make one. One solution was buying a smoothie—like "Apples and Greens" from Jamba Juice—though I had to be mindful that store-bought options (including bottled) can have a lot of sugar. That's when I started adding homemade versions into the rotation and realized how easy it was after all. If you still find yourself needing to go for the ready-made varieties, consider adding boosters like flax or chia seeds.

Now I get up earlier to make my own smoothies in my beloved Vitamix, which means I can control what kind of yummy goodness goes into my blends. (To this day, I add a teaspoon or tablespoon of turmeric to every smoothie I make to give an extra immune-system and cancer-fighting boost.) Before the Vitamix, my roommate Courtney and I had a juicer. We were inspired to juice by watching the documentary *Fat, Sick & Nearly Dead*, about a guy named Joe Cross who lost a hundred pounds by juicing. But the juicer was such a pain in the ass to take apart and put back together, we never used it. The Vitamix, on the other hand, is an amazing piece of machinery. So, before I get to my broke-girl smoothie suggestions, I'm going to make a case for splurging on a Vitamix.

Can I get all infomercial-y here for a minute? The Vitamix, a high-performance blender, will change your life and allow you to make healthy snacks, meals, and drinks like *that*. Seriously, break out the plastic for this. I'm telling you this as someone who used to choose foundation at the drug store not by color, but by whatever was the cheapest. Adam Shankman, a director and choreographer who produced *Hairspray, Rock of Ages,* and even the Oscars, told me to buy one, and I was like, "Shyeah right, Adam." But it's the best (financial) investment in my health that I've ever made. I use it for everything: soups, juices, smoothies, immunity elixirs, and even desserts.

I used to have a Target blender. It was a good start. But for someone who is super busy, a Vitamix cuts the prep time way down because there is no pre-chopping—just throw things in there whole! And you can make so much more than you would with Joe Blender. A normal blender is not able to blend a shit-ton of spices and things because it gets stopped up; a Vitamix takes literally thirty seconds to do the job. I'm not a huge fan of raw vegetables, so I can throw in broccoli, asparagus, and a bunch of spices and have soup for lunch in all of ten minutes.

The Vitamix is expensive—around $400. It costs basically $1 a day for a year, and you'll have it for the rest of your life (so it's a good thing you automatically get a lifetime warranty!). I just wish they had a little one that I could take on the road. Maybe they can call it Vitababy? I'm going to pitch it . . .

Anyway, every morning I walk into work with a mason jar full of smoothie. It's a joke on our set: "Beth, what's in your smoothie today?" "Well, we've got pineapple, spirulina . . . " But I have to say that Jennifer Coolidge rivals me in the smoothie department. She gets a gorgeous one every day from a place in her neighborhood. Mine always looks gross, like a cup of homemade brownish-green sludge. But that sludge is a winner! On any given day it's packed with immune-boosting, antioxidant-rich, hydrating, vitamin-packed goodness.

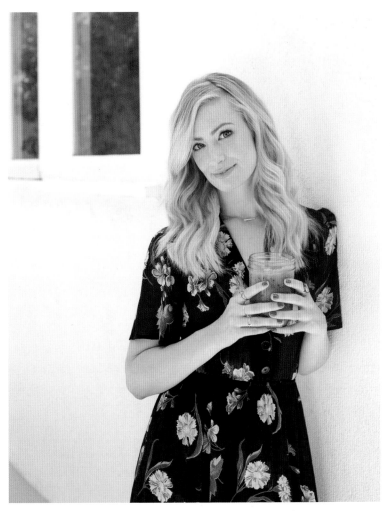

I'm just a girl, standing next to a wall, drinking a smoothie . . .

SMOOTHIE TIPS

- Cut up your fruits/veggies the night before and stash them in containers so you don't have to do prep work in the morning.
- Even though they're a little pricier, I recommend buying organic fruits and vegetables as often as you can. They're better for you, better for the environment, better for the farmer who grew them . . . and easier to clean. Just give them a good rinse before you begin chopping and dicing. If you're buying non-organic, give your produce a good wash with water and soap or a spritz of chemical-free produce wash. You can make your own with 2 cups cold tap water, ¼ cup distilled white vinegar, and 2 tablespoons lemon juice. Mix the ingredients and put them in a spray bottle. Then give your produce a couple of spritzes, let it sit for a minute, rinse it off with water, and you're good to go. Please note: The ingredients I use in the recipes that follow are all organic, unless noted otherwise.
- If your blender needs help blending, hit the "pulse" button a few times. Or some blenders/mixers come with a wand, which you can use to push everything down to the blades.
- Add a scoop of bee pollen (found at your local health food store) to any smoothie for energy-boosting B vitamins and allergy-symptom relief.
- Break a peeled banana into a few pieces, put the pieces in a plastic baggie, and throw it into the freezer. Use that for your smoothie the next morning to add creaminess, plus lots of chill without diluting the flavor.
- Add 1 teaspoon to 1 tablespoon (based on personal taste preference) coconut oil to any smoothie to boost absorption of the other nutrients in your drink.
- If things get sticky in your blender, scrape down the sides with a spatula and try blending again.
- Some of my recipes call for honey—the kind you get at the farmers' market is the best. If you buy fresh and local, you can also help ease allergies!
- All the smoothie recipes in this chapter make two small servings or one big one. Indulge according to your preference.
- Feel free to modify any of these recipes—either by making your own little tweaks or leaving things out that don't sound tasty to you. Or just use whatever you have in your fridge. These are basic suggestions and guidelines.

SMOOTHIES, DRINKS & SNACKS

"I DON'T LIKE SALAD ENOUGH, SO I'LL DRINK THIS INSTEAD" SMOOTHIE

Makes about 2 (8-ounce) servings

Here's a basic, great-way-to-start-your-day smoothie. The kale, spinach, celery, and cucumber offer the nutritional equivalent of jamming a salad into your cup, but the result doesn't taste too veggie-y because the fruit's sweetness counteracts the bitterness of the leafy greens. If you want a little more sweetness, boost the honey level. As for the berries, I like to buy them fresh and freeze them myself, but you can also grab them from the freezer section; frozen organic fruit is flash-frozen at its peak freshness, so it retains its vitamin content. Bon matin!

- ½ cup frozen blueberries
- ¼ cup raspberries
- 1 handful kale
- 2 big handfuls spinach
- ½ frozen banana (optional)
- 1 large rib celery
- ½ cucumber
- ½ thumb's worth fresh ginger
- 1 cup unsweetened almond milk, plus more if your smoothie gets too thick
- Dash of honey, or more to taste

Blend all that shiz together and enjoy!

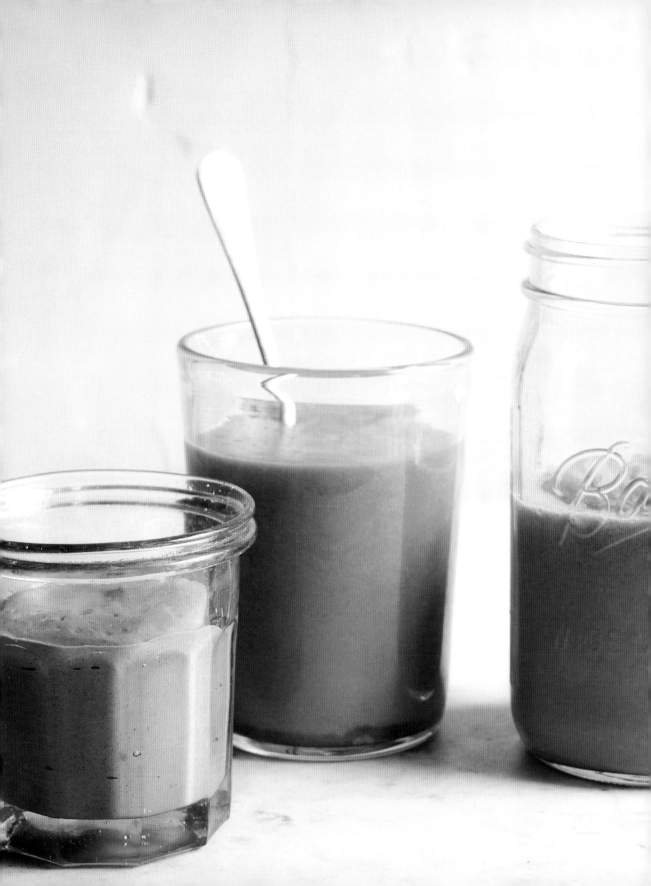

SMOOTH-OUT SMOOTHIE

Makes about 2 (8-ounce) servings

There are a few things I like about this smoothie: First of all, yum. The pineapple really counteracts the kale. Kale is SO GOOD FOR YOU, but it can taste bitter if you don't blend it with a sweet fruit (mango is another good option). Second, the blueberries are packed with antioxidants. And third, if you're feeling super bloated around your period, or you don't have the time (or the interest) to do 20 million crunches at the gym, it's nice to make a smoothie that counteracts belly bloat—there's an enzyme in pineapple that eases digestion and swelling!

  3 ounces nonfat Greek yogurt (plain, or vanilla for added sweetness)
  1 tablespoon almond butter
  ½ cup frozen blueberries
  ½ cup frozen pineapple
  1 cup kale
  ¾ cup water or 6 ice cubes for a thicker smoothie

Throw all the ingredients into a blender and blend until smooth.

VANILLA GREEN HEMP SEED SMOOTHIE

Makes about 2 (8-ounce) servings

This is an energizing way to start your day or give yourself a midday boost, especially with the vanilla hemp protein powder. I really like adding dates (without pits, of course) to any smoothie—they thicken things up and sweeten the blend with a healthier kind of sugar. Also, the coconut water—a recent staple for me, especially in the morning—is super hydrating. The hemp seeds are a great source of essential fatty acids, protein, and vitamin E, and the Greek yogurt is going to give you some protein and a probiotic boost.

¾ cup coconut water
1 cup packed spinach leaves
½ cup plain Greek yogurt
1 cup frozen mango chunks
1 large frozen banana
2 small pitted dates
1 tablespoon raw, shelled hemp seeds
2 tablespoons chia seeds
1 (1-inch) piece fresh ginger, peeled
2 tablespoons vanilla hemp protein powder

Toss all the ingredients into a blender and blend until smooth. (Remember, if your blender needs a little help incorporating everything, use the pulse button.)

SORT-OF SHERBET SMOOTHIE

Makes about 2 (8-ounce) servings

This is the perfect smoothie for summertime, when you're sitting around the pool and the kids are having popsicles and you're having a fruity/sherbet kind of craving. A handful of strawberries has more vitamin C than an entire orange—so it's good protection against summer colds, too! Speaking of C, the amount of vitamin C in baobab powder, made from baobab fruit from Africa, puts both oranges and strawberries to shame. A total superfood, it's also packed with minerals like calcium, copper, iron, magnesium, potassium, and zinc. If its sour taste bugs you, add a little honey to counteract it. And if you're not familiar with goji berries, try them out. They're an excellent antioxidant and a great source of beta-carotene. If you want to make this smoothie a little more filling, you can add a little whey or rice protein powder.

1½ cups frozen strawberries
1 cup sliced frozen banana (about 2 small bananas)
2 tablespoons freshly squeezed lemon juice (about 1 lemon)
6 ice cubes
1 teaspoon baobab powder (look for it online if you can't find it in your store)
1 teaspoon dried goji berries (optional; substitute for baobab if it's unavailable)
2 to 3 tablespoons whey or rice protein powder (optional)

Toss all the ingredients into a blender and blend until smooth.

GO-FOR-GREEN SMOOTHIE

Makes about 2 (8-ounce) servings

My friend Tyler, who I worked with at the Geffen (remember, the playhouse where I bartended?), introduced me to green drinks. When I asked him to remind me how we got on the topic, he said:

After a trip to Subway where you got a meatball sub . . . we were discussing your diet being similar to that of a ten-year-old boy. It was funny, but things got weird when you said that you don't eat vegetables. Like, at all. Everyone kept trying to give you recipes or ideas for snacks, but you weren't into it. So I told you about these bottled green smoothies you could buy at the grocery store, but when I listed the ingredients, I'm pretty sure you threw up in your mouth a little. Long story short: I convinced you it tasted like rainbows and apple juice, so you eventually tried it and liked it. And then you drank it every day for a long time. I didn't tell you that you were consuming a huge amount of sugar . . . I figured, whatevs, at least it's not as bad as the time you were addicted to Sudafed for a year! But I digress.

Well, it's true. Eventually I replaced the store-bought, sugar-dressed-up-as-vegetables smoothies with this green juice inspired by a recipe from Gather & Feast. It is packed with all kinds of nutrients like vitamins A and K, iron, and beta-carotene. And believe me, it tastes like rainbows and apple juice. (PS: Once I started drinking these smoothies and cutting a lot of dairy out of my diet, my constant need for Sudafed to ease sinus symptoms also became a thing of the past.)

- 1 green apple
- 1 cucumber
- 1 rib celery
- ½ pear
- 1 (1-centimeter) piece fresh ginger, peeled and grated
- 2 tablespoons chia seeds
- Juice of ½ lime
- ½ cup water
- 1 cup ice
- 1 large handful baby spinach
- 1 handful kale (about 6 small leaves)

Add everything but the ice and leafy greens to a blender. Blend away, then add the ice and pulse to combine. Finally, add the leafy greens and blend until smooth.

HOPPIN' JALAPEÑO SMOOTHIE

Makes about 2 (8-ounce) servings

I love this smoothie, which comes from Kris Carr of *Crazy Sexy Cancer* fame. I'm a big spice fanatic, so this smoothie hits the spot. The crisp apple along with the jalapeño—yum! It's like a G-rated margarita with nutritional value . . . you can't ask for more.

- 1 handful spinach
- 2 apples, chopped
- 1 cucumber, chopped
- ½ jalapeño pepper, chopped (remove seeds if you want less heat)
- Juice of 1 lime
- 1 tablespoon hemp protein powder
- 1 cup water
- 1 cup ice

Toss all the ingredients into a blender and blend until smooth.

> Be careful when handling jalapeño seeds, as they can make your fingers (and anything you touch) sting badly. Consider wearing plastic gloves to keep yourself protected.

CHOCOCADO SMOOTHIE

Makes about 2 (8-ounce) servings

During summertime when I was a kid, my family used to ride our bikes to get ice cream after dinner. To this day, when the weather is lovely I still crave that sweet treat. Who isn't always craving chocolate? Luckily, this smoothie tastes like a chocolate milk shake, with the bonus of healthy fat from the avocado. There are a million chocolate-avocado smoothie recipes out there; I think this one from Thrive Market is the best of the best, so I just tweaked it a tiny bit. Toss a little spinach in there for the extra nutrition boost—you'll never taste it.

- 2 tablespoons raw cacao powder
- ½ ripe avocado
- ½ frozen banana
- 2 tablespoons almond butter
- 1 handful spinach leaves
- 3 pitted dates
- 1 tablespoon hemp, chia, or flax seeds
- Dash of cinnamon
- 2 teaspoons vanilla extract
- 1 cup unsweetened almond milk
- ½ cup crushed ice

Put the cacao powder, avocado, banana, almond butter, spinach, dates, seeds, cinnamon, and vanilla in a blender. Pour in almond milk and crushed ice. Blend until smooth.

MUST-HAVE MINT SMOOTHIE

Makes about 2 (8-ounce) servings

Another delicious dessert-style smoothie, with a great creamy consistency from the cashews. Cashews will keep you full, so if you're in the "I need a smoothie for lunch" zone, try this recipe.

 1 frozen banana, broken into thirds
 2 handfuls spinach
 1 to 2 tablespoons cacao nibs, or more to taste
 2 to 3 fresh mint leaves, or more to taste
Dash of honey or agave
 1 cup unsweetened almond milk, plus more if your smoothie gets too thick
10 cashews, plus more if you want a creamier smoothie

Toss all the ingredients into a blender and blend until smooth.

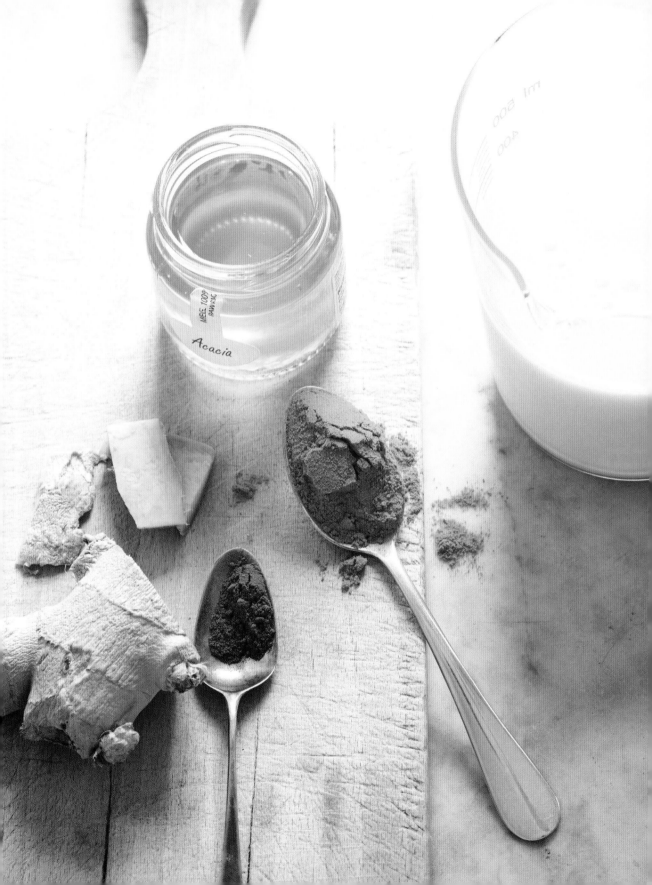

TURMERIC TEA

Makes 4 small teacup servings or 2 mugfuls

I love starting my day with this tea because turmeric has excellent anti-inflammatory and antioxidant properties, and the spices warm you right up. I especially get a yen for it when the weather cools and cold/flu season starts strolling in. And when I think a cold is coming on, I make this tea. A few cups later, I feel fine. Can't prove it in court, but I'm saying it's the healing power of turmeric tea. And the cayenne is also a winner when you're under the weather—it clears those sinuses right up. If you wanna be a real badass, you can add a thumbnail's worth of minced fresh ginger—but you have to mean business, because the taste is INTENSE.

2 cups nondairy milk (I prefer unsweetened coconut milk, but any nut milk will do)
1 teaspoon ground turmeric
½ teaspoon ground cinnamon
1 teaspoon honey or agave
Thumbnail's worth minced fresh ginger (optional)
Pinch of cayenne pepper (optional)

Put all the ingredients in a blender and blend until smooth. Pour into a saucepan over medium and heat until hot but not boiling (about 3 to 5 minutes). Pour into teacups or mugs and drink while it's hot.

SMALL BUT POWERFUL: WATER

Drink water—lots of it. I know that's like a crazy Hollywood thing to say, but could Cameron Diaz, Beyoncé, Jennifer Aniston, AND me really all be wrong? (Jen's beauty advice: "Drink water, stay hydrated, and sleep. It's so boring, yet so simple." Love her.) As the Mayo Clinic explains: "Water is your body's principal chemical component and makes up about 60 percent of your body weight. Every system in your body depends on water. For example, water flushes toxins out of vital organs, carries nutrients to your cells, and provides a moist [yuck] environment for ear, nose and throat tissues." Without water (and other hydrating fluids like unsweetened nut milks or juices, coconut water, or decaf tea), your energy drains and your system slows down.

Drinking water isn't easy for me because for years I couldn't have just plain water (maybe I'd drink some bottled water here or there). I wanted flavor. I was a sodaholic my whole life. I loved it. So if I was thirsty, that's what I drank. Plus, I have the bladder of an eighty-year-old woman, so drinking extra water just makes it ten times worse. My friends think I have a bladder problem. They're like, "You need to be on medication." I say, "I am thirty years old, I am not going to be on medication." They'll just have to learn to love my mini-bladder. Really, I think it's genetic. If you go on a vacation with my family, you'll soon realize that we all have to stop all the time to pee. We pretty much can't get a half hour down the road without having a bathroom break. And on set, I Kegel the hell out of myself until they say "Cut!" . . . in my seven-inch heels, trying not to fall backwards. It's TMI but it's true.

So initially, to wean myself off diet-carbonated-who-knows-what and increase my H_2O intake, I started drinking LaCroix carbonated water. It's infused with fruit and tastes like soda. Then I cut back on coffee. I used to guzzle it in order to avoid the sudden drop in energy I'd have in the afternoons after eating a ton of sugar, but I noticed that the more water and green tea I drank on show nights, the less likely I was to crash. Now, if I really need the caffeine, I get it from black breakfast tea instead, which is gentler on my body and not as dehydrating as coffee. My other afternoon energy reboot used to be milk shakes. I mean, they're hydrating, right? Not exactly. The water/green tea combo hits the spot, so I don't even miss milk shakes. (And I loooooved them—Michael Patrick King, my boss, once had to grab one out of my hand while we were shooting.)

I try to drink a total of two liters of water, smoothies, or tea daily. You often hear the stat that you should be drinking six to eight 8-ounce glasses of water a day, but not everyone can manage it. Nutritionist Maya Feller says: "I usually tell my well patients to drink to thirst. There is a fine line between being thirsty (which usually means you are mildly dehydrated), and being aware that it's time to have a glass of water. Don't wait until you are thirsty. Instead, hydrate yourself at regular intervals throughout the day. A great indicator of hydration is your output. Yes, the color of your urine will tell you a lot. If your urine is a dark color and you are not taking medications or supplements, that could be an indicator of dehydration. If your urine is clear like water, you may be drinking too much. The happy medium is a pale yellow." So check your pee and go to town!

The easiest way to drink more water? Always have some around! As in, a reusable water bottle that you can throw in your bag, car, etc. My favorite ones are the forty-ounce big guys from Klean Kanteen. I bring them to work and try to drink at least two full bottles when I'm shooting. The reason I'm a Klean Kanteen fan? First of all, they contain no BPA, phthalates, lead, or other toxins—not all bottles can claim that (especially plastic ones). Also, they don't retain or impart flavors, so my water always tastes fresh. Finally, they are easy to clean—I mean, *klean*. I'm also a big fan of S'well bottles, which are seventeen ounces and come in a variety of gorgeous colors and patterns. They can keep your drink cold for twenty-four hours or hot for twelve, so they're great for carting around tea with lemon when I'm under the weather, or keeping some refreshing cool water with me when I'm out carousing at night.

Keep your bottle close and sip, sip, sip. And if you need to give your intake a boost, make yourself drink a full glass when you first wake up in the morning, or before or after you exercise. Add a glass to your meals (replacing soda or juice) and make sure you drink it all. Think of it as free medicine from Mother Nature.

WATER TIP

Drink a glass of water fifteen minutes before you plan to eat.
It will hydrate your digestive track and help your intestines
absorb nutrients from your chow.

SNACKS

Okay, you are now a skilled beverage-ist (and you probably pee twenty times a day, like I do). You have every reason to feel confident about moving on to a new level of improved eating. Here are some sound snack ideas, no cooking required.

Tips & Tricks for Good Snacking

Get nutty. Almonds are my saving grace. I keep them in the glove compartment of my car and in my dressing room. Raw peanuts, too, in the shell. They're fun to peel and *sooo* delicious. Yes, nuts are a high-fat food, so don't go crazy with them (a handful, or about twenty nuts, is a decent serving). But that fat keeps you feeling full and satiated, which might prevent you from sniffing around for processed junk food. And ironically, studies have shown that eating nuts can lower heart disease. Almonds happen to be chock-full of vitamin E, magnesium, and potassium. Whole almonds with their skins intact seem to have the greatest health benefits. So enjoy!

Replace potato with popcorn-o. I am a crazy potato chip addict. I freakin' crave their salty, crunchy deliciousness, especially when I'm on set, all stressed and running around. Crunch = comfort. But popcorn is a better alternative to chips because it's loaded with fiber. Fiber not only makes you feel fuller, but also more satisfied, because it digests slowly. Popcorn lightbulb! It's still salty and crunchy, but it's waaaay better for me. I now keep bags of butter-free popcorn in my dressing room. BAM. PS: I also sometimes top my tomato soup with a heaping pile of popcorn. It sounds weird, but it's DELISH and makes me feel fuller than just eating the soup alone.

Care to crunch? It's always good to have some fresh fruit and vegetables handy so that you're not tempted to grab whatever junk is lurking in your pantry/desk drawer/office vending machine. There finally came a time when I—gasp—found myself craving good, fresh produce for a snack instead of like, Rice Krispies treats. Those snacks include carrots and hummus, cut-up red bell peppers, and sugar snap peas. On the fruit side, I grab something easy and filling like an apple, a peach, or a pear. Plus, it's easy these days to find fresh yet cheap produce (for example, at your local farmers' market or Trader Joe's).

Take the cake. Not the sheet cake, silly, the rice cake. Make sure you have a stash of unsalted brown rice cakes and almond butter available at all times. A little bit sweet, a little bit crunchy, and very filling. This snack also gives you a boost of energy when you hit that late-afternoon slump or you need some pre-workout zest.

See? Easy-peasy and yummy. And here's a quick shopping list for snacks you can pick up next time you're at the store . . . all things you can grab from the shelf or prepare without cooking. That way, you never need to turn to that roll of chocolate chip cookie dough in your fridge—go ahead and throw that out, by the way.

Ten (Okay, Eleven) Snacks to Have in Your House at All Times

- Unsalted brown rice cakes
- Almond butter (try Justin's all-natural version)
- Red bell peppers
- Unsalted popcorn
- Almonds
- Baby carrots
- Hummus
- Blueberries or grapes
- Sugar snap peas or celery sticks
- Pumpkin seeds
- Greek yogurt

HAPPY TRAIL (MIXES)!

Another great snack to have on hand at all times is your favorite trail mix. You can mix and blend nuts, seeds, dried fruits, and even a little bit of sweetness like carob chips or granola to your heart's content. Here's a general formula that's easy to follow:

50% nuts
25% dried fruit
25% seeds & stuff (see below)
And a sprinkle of "just for fun," less than 1 tablespoon (see below)

Select from the following and make your own!

- **NUTS (raw, unsalted, and shelled):** almonds, Brazil nuts, cashews, hazelnuts, pistachios, macadamias, pecans, peanuts
- **DRIED FRUIT (sans added sugar):** apples, blueberries, bananas, cherries, cranberries, dates, figs, pineapple, mango, raisins
- **SEEDS & STUFF:** pumpkin seeds, sunflower seeds, flax seeds, sesame seeds, hemp seeds, goji berries
- **JUST FOR FUN:** chocolate or carob chips, cacao nibs, air-popped popcorn, pretzels, yogurt-covered raisins, cereal (such as Chex or puffed rice), flaked coconut, granola, wasabi peas, candied ginger bits. If you really insist on candy like M&M's or mini-marshmallows, keep them to a tablespoon or less.

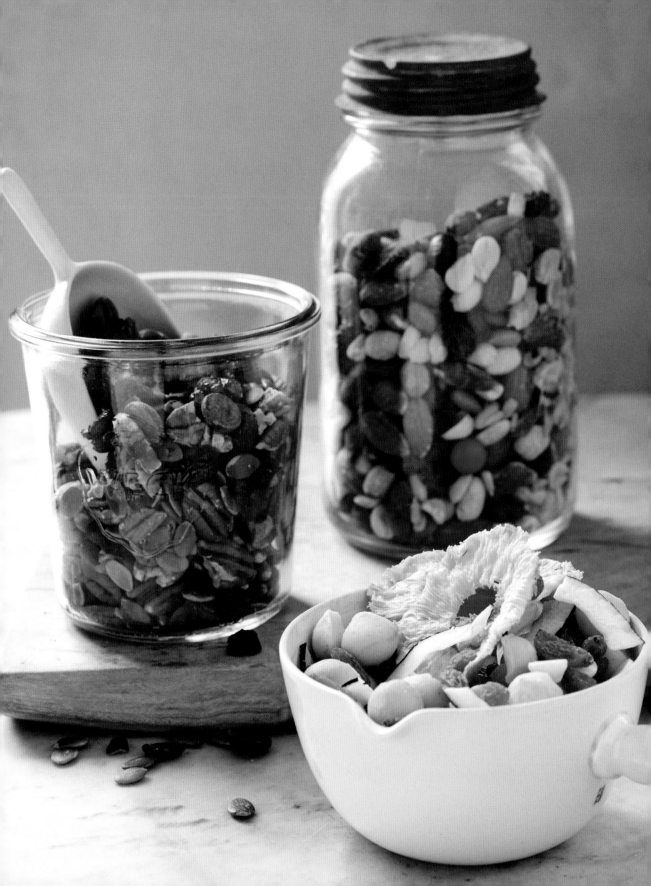

SOME OF MY FAVORITE TRAIL MIXES

HAPPY TRAILS (A TWIST ON "GORP," OR "GOOD OLD RAISINS & PEANUTS")

- 50% peanuts and almonds
- 25% raisins
- 25% sunflower seeds
- 1 tablespoon M&M's

FALL FLAVOR

- 50% pecans
- 25% cranberries
- 25% pumpkin seeds
- 1 tablespoon chocolate or carob chips

SUNSHINE MIX

- 50% macadamia nuts
- 25% golden raisins and pineapple
- 25% sunflower seeds
- 1 tablespoon white chocolate chips
- 1 tablespoon flaked coconut

INSTEAD OF THIS . . . TRY THIS!

BOWL OF CHIPS	➤	BOWL OF POPCORN
SNICKERS BAR	➤	RICE CAKE WITH ALMOND BUTTER, SPRINKLED WITH CACAO NIBS
CHEESE & CRACKERS	➤	CARROTS & HUMMUS (page 67 or store-bought)
BOWL OF ICE CREAM	➤	BOWL OF GREEK YOGURT WITH HONEY DRIZZLE
BAG OF PRETZELS	➤	BAG OF HOMEMADE TRAIL MIX

EAT BEAUTIFULLY

Good food isn't just good for you on the inside—it can make you beautiful, too. I learned so much about "beauty foods" from the book *Eat Pretty: Nutrition for Beauty, Inside and Out*, written by beauty editor and certified health coach Jolene Hart. In fact, her wisdom is so major that I rang her up and asked her a few questions of my own.

Jolene, what are your favorite beauty superfoods, and why?
I think lemons are incredible beauty superfoods, and I consume lemon juice and sometimes the organic pith and peel daily, whether in warm lemon water, homemade dressings, or smoothies. Lemon juice is highly alkaline, cleansing to the body and the digestive tract, and loaded with collagen-building vitamin C. I'm obsessed with avocados and probably eat a whole one every day, which my skin loves for the healthy fats and my body loves for the instant energy. Leafy greens are such nutrient-dense foods for beauty, with tons of the skin-smoothing, healing vitamin A and the antioxidant vitamin C, plus bonus beauty minerals, so I make sure to eat at least one serving daily. And foods that contain natural probiotics, like raw sauerkraut or other fermented veggies, are fantastic for a healthy gut, which reflects in clear, radiant skin.

How can I work seeds like flax, hemp, and pumpkin into my diet?
My view is, where can you *not* add seeds?! Seeds like flax, hemp, and pumpkin are so packed with skin-loving fats, beauty minerals, blood sugar–stabilizing fiber, and often extra protein, that an extra scoop or sprinkle is such an easy beauty boost for a meal. And they work in both sweet and savory foods. My smoothies always have seeds, and my salads (both green salads and grain salads) do, too, for texture and flavor. I also love adding them to a homemade dressing (blend it up for extra creaminess) and as a base for raw truffles and crusts.

What are the most hydrating foods I can eat? Drinks I can drink?
Your skin is 70 percent water, so hydration is super important for keeping it looking its best. Opt for water-rich fruits and veggies (your body absorbs their moisture slowly as you digest them) like cucumber, watermelon, apples, zucchini, peppers, melons—there are so many. And help your skin lock in that moisture by

eating plenty of healthy fats like coconut, raw nuts and seeds, avocado, and wild salmon. Sipping pure water or lemon or lime water is amazing for hydration, but herbal teas also do the trick, and coconut water is amazing for hydration with the added benefit of electrolyte balance.

What foods are best for my skin?
In truth, only you can answer that. Practice listening to your body and seeing how you react to certain foods to figure out how they affect your unique body. In general, opt for foods that are naturally colorful (color signals the presence of antiaging phytochemicals that hold amazing power for your skin), nutrient dense (fresh vegetables pack in amazing nutritional benefits in relatively small servings), and seasonal (to target the shifting needs of your beauty and body throughout the year). Also, make sure you're keeping your blood sugar steady with ample protein and healthy fats at each meal, and you'll keep your skin happy, too.

I know you're not a fan of sugar, so what do you eat when you want a sweet treat?
I'm not a fan of what sugar does to my skin, but I definitely save room for dessert when it's special, and when I really can't resist. My sweet tooth is something I continually work to balance! Day to day, I stick to dark chocolate or carob (I've loved the taste since I was a kid, and there's no caffeine to worry about), home-made truffles (raw nuts, seeds, raw cacao powder, maple syrup, dates, etc., blended up in a food processor), or even sweet smoothies with coconut milk, fruit, and cinnamon for blood sugar stability. I also love to bake fruit crumbles with a topping of gluten-free oats, flaked coconut, cinnamon and ginger, and a little coconut sugar. Since I shifted my diet to include more protein and healthy fats, though, I don't feel as controlled by sugar cravings, and I'm able to pass up sweets when my body or skin is showing signs that I've indulged a bit too much. It's all about balance, without feeling restriction.

Isn't Jolene amazing? Based on her advice, as well as my own experimentation, here's a list of my favorite things to eat that help you look as good on the outside as you feel on the inside. I realize you can't throw all the foods listed below into a smoothie or turn them into a snack (I mean, if you can handle a garlic smoothie, go for it), but you'll find many of these foods in the following chapters of the book.

Fruits and veggies: Eating fruits and veggies hydrates you, making your skin look plumper and fresher. And studies have shown that eating these foods makes us look more attractive to others because they alter the hue and glow of our complexions.

Green/string beans: These contain a lot of silicon, which keeps your skin, hair, and nails flexible and strong (just stay away from too many gel manicures). Keep a cooked batch in your fridge for easy-to-pack snacks.

Flax seeds: Flax seeds are full of omega-3s that reduce inflammation, which can help with things like sore muscles and joints and also skin inflammation like rashes. They also aid in oil production for skin, leading to better hydration and causing fewer blackheads and a healthier scalp. Put some in your smoothies or on your cereal.

Hemp seeds/hemp protein powder: Like flax seeds, hemp seeds and hemp protein powder are packed with omega-3s, which are very good for your skin, especially for healing eczema. They're also a good source of iron and zinc, helpful for fighting off colds (see the Vanilla Green Hemp Seed Smoothie recipe on page 45).

Almond milk: Well, you know I loves me my almonds and unsweetened almond milk (I drink unsweetened to avoid added sugars). It's not just that it tastes delish—a cup of unsweetened almond milk includes a daily dose of vitamin E that keeps skin moisturized and protected from the sun. Drink it straight, add it to tea or smoothies, or pour it over cereal or oatmeal.

Spinach: I'm a huge fan of spinach for health reasons, and for beauty reasons, too: It's a great source of calcium, which is essential for strong teeth and nails. The vitamin A in spinach contributes to making skin glow. If you're not up for a big bowl, sneak it into recipes and smoothies and you'll barely be able to taste it.

Pumpkin seeds: Check out my Zesty Toasted Pumpkin Seeds recipe on page 69. Super tasty, super good for you, and a beauty booster, too: These seeds are full of iron, which supports strong, shiny nails. (Also try lentils and oats for extra iron.)

Garlic: I like garlic for a million reasons, but did you know that the sulfur in garlic supports healthy hair? True dat. Also, allicin, the phytochemical that gives garlic that zingy taste and smell, slows the formation of wrinkles.

Blueberries: Another food that's easy to eat on the go—while doing your beauty a good deed. Eating blueberries boosts skin elasticity, protects against damage from the sun, and defends against wrinkles. No wonder they're called a superfood.

EATING BEAUTIFULLY TIP

In case you needed any more reasons to avoid excess sugar . . . just remember that sugar breaks down collagen, which directly contributes to wrinkles, age spots, and, of course, cellulite.

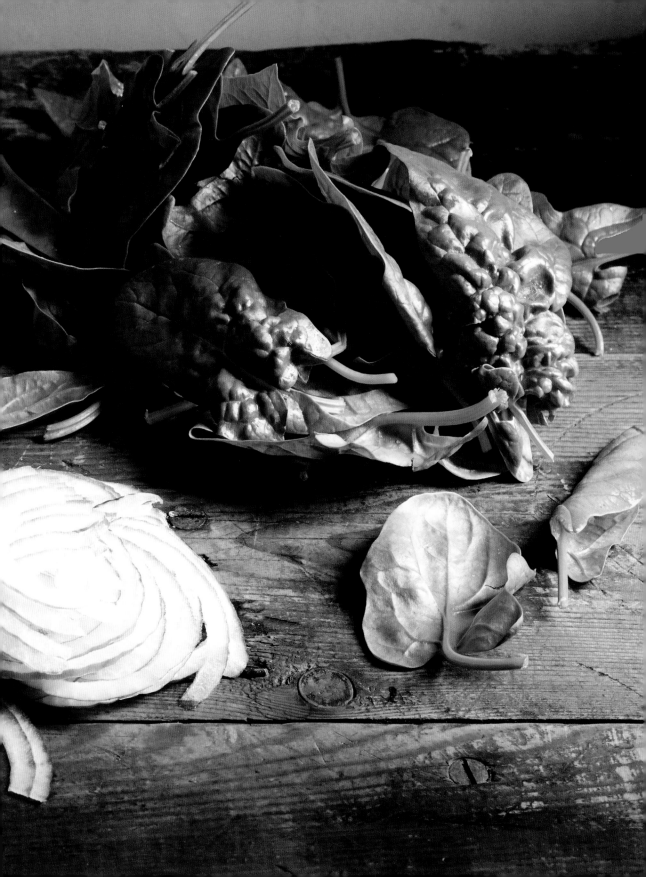

CHAPTER 4

THE "S" SECTION:
SPREADS, STARTERS, SALADS & SIDES

It's time to kick things up a notch and start making some stuff—and not just throwing a bunch of things in a blender. You can easily make a spread or starter of your own to build on your healthy-eating goals and to make your taste buds go *YES!* My go-tos in this chapter are hummus, almond butter, and "almost cheese" (it's amazing, and trust me, I'm a cheese-aholic). These are quick and easy recipes, and you'll know right away if you need to start over (unlike waiting for a main dish to come out of the oven). But I'm pretty sure you'll be able to get these right on the first try.

These recipes are not only great as appetizers, light meals, and snacks, they're also perfect for feeding a crowd, which I've put to the test because Michael and I love to have people over. We throw Fourth of July parties, Halloween pumpkin-carving events, Thanksgiving dinners, you name it. Kat and I even started a book club with sixteen other girls. It's called "The Grape Expectations Literary Society," and it's become our favorite thing to do every month. Lately we've read *Luckiest Girl Alive, Blackout*, and *Cold Comfort Farm*, and we're about to start in on *My Brilliant Friend*. Kat even designed merch for the book club members, and let's just say that a monocle makes an appearance. Nerd alert!

SPREADS & STARTERS

YUMMY HUMMUS

Makes about 1½ cups

This spread/snack is a staple for me because it's so delish and filling, due to all the fiber in the chickpeas. Once you make this recipe, you will never get store-bought again—it's that good (and easy). It calls for the ingredient tahini, or sesame seed paste. If you don't know where in the store to find it, just ask—I was too embarrassed and it took me forever to zero in on it! But you can't be shy when it comes to your health. Bonus: Tahini is full of zinc, which helps keep your skin clear.

1 (15-ounce) can chickpeas (a.k.a. garbanzo beans), drained
½ cup plus 2 tablespoons extra-virgin olive oil
2 tablespoons tahini
Juice and zest of ½ lemon
Salt, to taste
Sprinkle of cayenne pepper or paprika
Chopped fresh parsley, for garnish
4 (6-inch) pitas, each cut into 6 wedges, or sliced bell peppers and carrot sticks, for serving

Combine all the ingredients except parsley in a blender and blend until smooth. Adjust the seasoning if needed and garnish with parsley. Serve with pita bread or sliced bell peppers and carrot sticks.

MAKE IT YOUR OWN:

I toss a little jalapeño into my hummus for an extra-spicy kick.

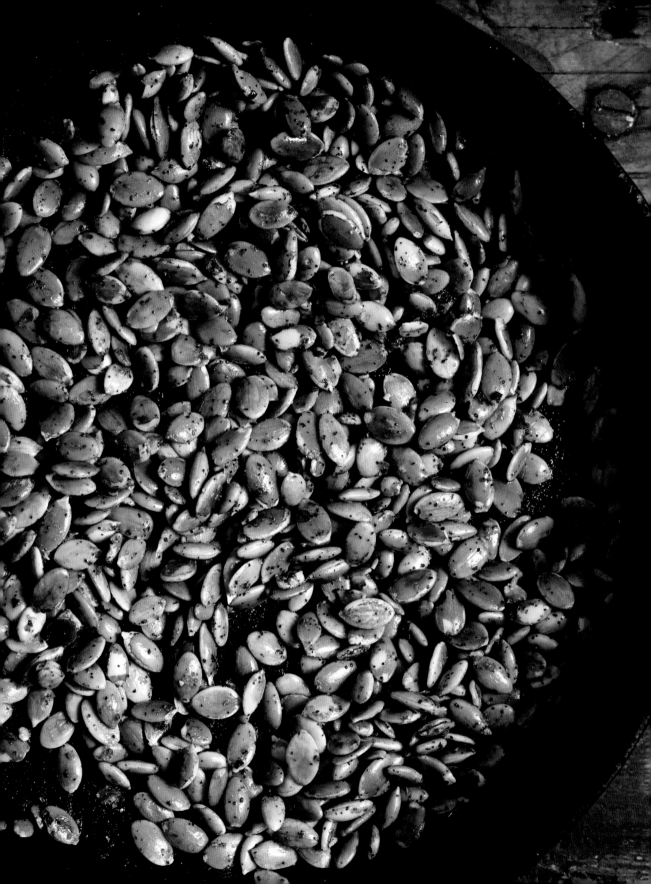

ZESTY TOASTED PUMPKIN SEEDS

Makes about 1 cup

I'm a big fan of seeds—sunflower, chia, flax. But it's pumpkin seeds that always remind me of good family times as a kid, carving pumpkins and toasting the seeds to eat when the job was done. In addition to being a tasty snack when you're craving crunch, pumpkin seeds are packed with zinc, which is excellent for fighting colds in autumnal weather. You can stash them in a plastic baggie or a mason jar, and they should stay fresh for about a week. But you'll probably eat them up long before that.

- 1 cup raw unsalted pumpkin seeds
- 1 tablespoon canola oil
- 1 teaspoon sugar
- ½ teaspoon ground cumin
- ½ teaspoon chipotle powder
- ¼ teaspoon kosher salt
- ¼ teaspoon ground cinnamon
- Pinch of cayenne pepper

Place the pumpkin seeds in a large skillet over medium heat. Cook for 4 minutes, or until toasted, stirring constantly (the seeds will pop slightly as they toast).

Combine the canola oil and remaining ingredients in a large bowl. Add the seeds, tossing to coat. Arrange the seeds in a single layer on a paper towel–lined baking sheet and let them cool for 10 minutes.

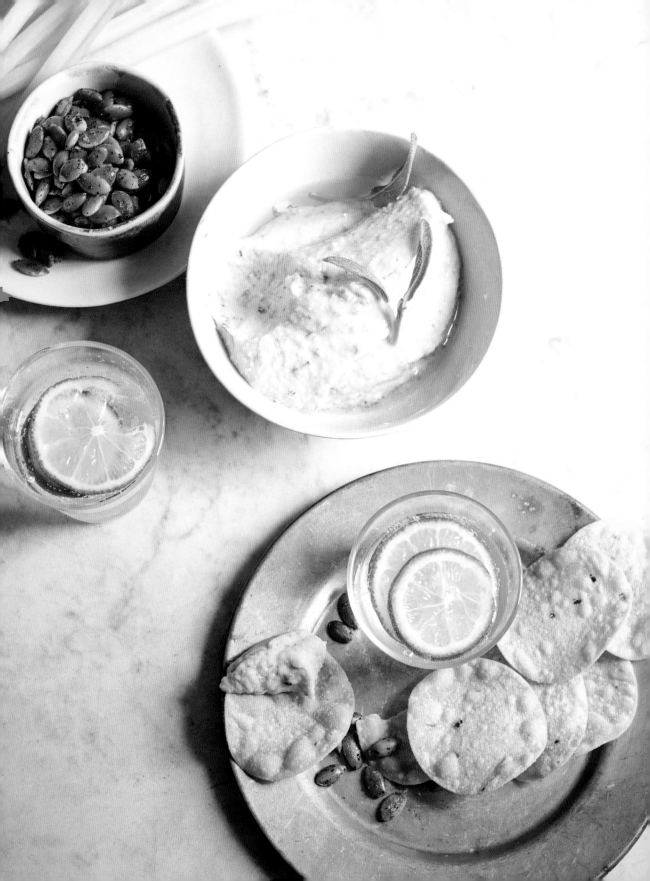

WHITE BEAN DIP
WITH ROSEMARY AND SAGE

Makes about 1½ cups

I love to make this recipe from *Cooking Light* for my book club girls when they come over. It's tasty and a little bit sophisticated, with fresh herbs like sage and rosemary, which always make me really happy. Plus, beans are a great source of fiber and protein—fantastic if you're not eating a lot of meat.

You could put this out with some pita wedges, or my favorite, sliced red and yellow bell peppers. They're sturdy enough for scooping and look gorgeous.

- 2 tablespoons freshly squeezed lemon juice
- 1 tablespoon extra-virgin olive oil
- 2 teaspoons minced fresh rosemary
- 2 teaspoons minced fresh sage, plus a full sprig for garnish (optional)
- ¼ teaspoon freshly ground black pepper
- 2 garlic cloves, chopped
- 1 (19-ounce) can cannellini beans or other white beans, drained and rinsed
- 4 (6-inch) pitas, each cut into 6 wedges, or sliced veggies, for serving

Combine everything but the pita and sprig of sage in a blender and blend until smooth. Garnish with sage sprig and serve with pita or veggies.

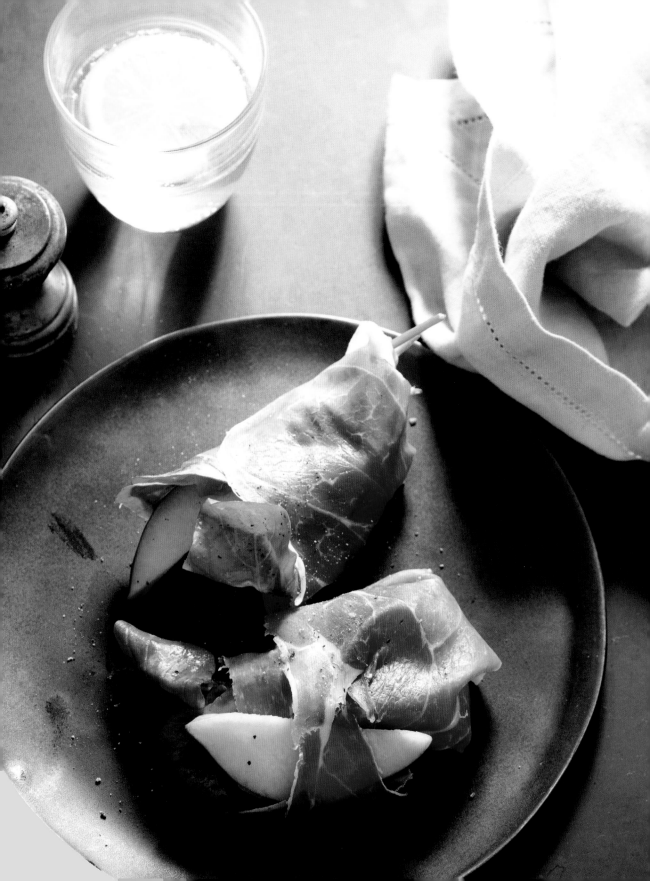

NECTARINE & ARUGULA ROLLS

Makes 12 servings

This light dish is perfect for entertaining when the weather is toasty. It's quick and simple to make, and it's a real crowd-pleaser—easy to pick up with your hands and eat. It's a nice combo of sweet and tart because the sweetness of the fruit contrasts nicely with the bitterness of the arugula. And somehow those flavors totally work with prosciutto, a kind of sweet meat. Now, I love prosciutto, but it's a cured meat, so I try to eat it in moderation because there's some proof that eating too much processed meat can increase your chances of some forms of cancer. If you're not a prosciutto fan or if you prefer to make a vegetarian version of this starter, try slices of Swiss, provolone, or muenster cheese instead (added bonus: calcium!).

   4 cups lightly packed arugula leaves
   1 teaspoon extra-virgin olive oil
  ⅛ teaspoon freshly ground black pepper
  12 (½-ounce) slices prosciutto, halved lengthwise
   3 nectarines (about ¾ pound), each cut into 8 wedges

Combine the arugula, olive oil, and pepper in a large bowl and toss gently to mix. Arrange 3 or 4 arugula leaves at one end of a prosciutto strip. Place a nectarine wedge on top of the arugula and roll that sucker up. Put the entire bundle, seam-side down, on a serving plate. Repeat with the remaining arugula, prosciutto, and nectarines.

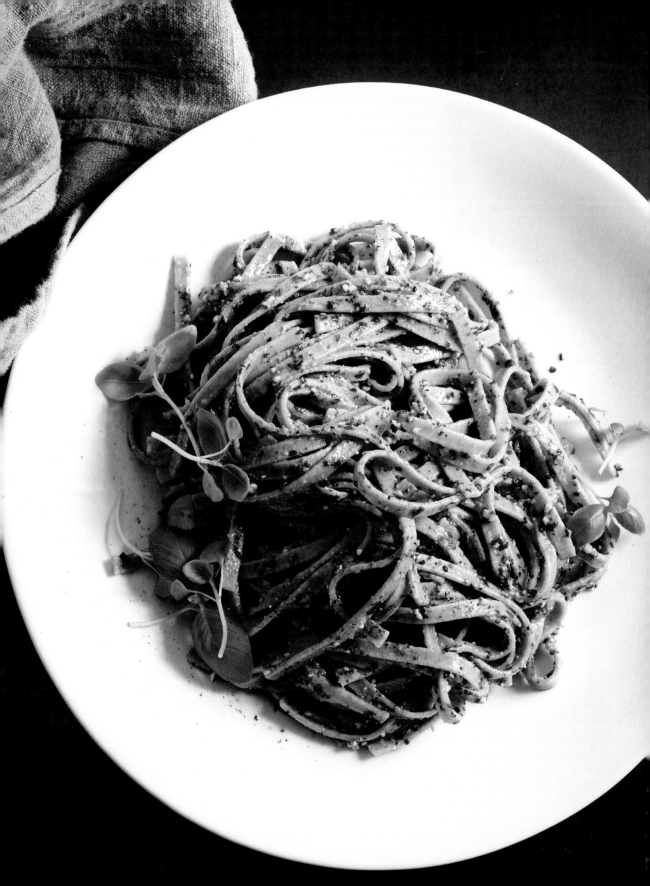

PESTO SAUCE

Makes about 1 cup

My favorite way to eat pesto—a green sauce traditionally made with basil, garlic, pine nuts, olive oil, and Parmesan—is on pasta, but it's also delish on veggies. You can drizzle it on broccoli, zucchini, peppers—you name it. (Veggies can be so boring—you gotta amp 'em up!) This pesto recipe is super easy and quick to make, and you can toss it on cold pasta for a delicious pesto salad. It was a big hit at our Fourth of July BBQ last year . . .

½ cup olive oil
½ cup grated Parmesan cheese
3 medium garlic cloves
2 cups fresh basil leaves
3 tablespoons pine nuts
Pinch of red pepper flakes (optional)
Salt and freshly ground black pepper, to taste

Put all the ingredients except salt and pepper into a blender and blend on medium-high speed. Season to taste with salt and pepper. Store the pesto in a glass jar in your fridge, where it will keep for about a week. Or you can freeze it for up to a few months.

FREEZING TIP:

Pour your pesto into an ice cube tray before you freeze it, and store the tray in a plastic bag. Anytime you need an individual serving, just pop out a pesto cube and heat it up.

BETH'S EASY ALMOND BUTTER

Makes about 2 cups

Almond butter is a staple for me at work because I rarely have time to sit down and eat a full meal—and I need lots of energy while I'm on the job. I love to schmear it on brown rice cakes or toasted whole wheat bread. It's a great snack for when you're on the run—and very easy to sneak in in between appointments when you're stuck on the 405. Cut up an apple or grab a few rice cakes and spread on the almond butter, then pack them in a container to keep with you in the car or at your desk. Also, you can add almond butter to smoothies for a thicker texture and a richer taste. And the best part? It's so easy to make!

¼ cup canola oil
4 cups roasted unsalted almonds

Put the oil in a high-powered blender (preferably a Vitamix), along with 1 cup of almonds at a time. Blend on high. Keep adding almonds, 1 cup at a time, until all 4 cups have been added. Blend until creamy.

Store the almond butter in an airtight container in the fridge for up to 3 months (the oil will separate, but just stir everything back together). It can also be frozen for longer storage.

VEGAN "ALMOST CHEESE" SAUCE

Makes 2 cups

So, it's Super Bowl Sunday and you've got a crowd of vegans headed over to your house. They're going to love this—and you will, too. Okay, it doesn't taste EXACTLY like melted cheese, as the consistency isn't quite as creamy, but you kind of get addicted to it. Plus, you have the option of adding some heat to it to give it a little more depth of flavor. So on game day, when you're ready to add cheese to just about everything, break out this recipe. Drizzle it over chips or serve it as a dip for veggies or toasted pita. Or, if you're craving mac and cheese (who isn't?), you can stir this "almost cheese" sauce into whole wheat or gluten-free brown rice pasta shells to make a healthier version.

This recipe includes an ingredient called nutritional yeast, which is a little different than the yeast you use in most baking recipes. It gives foods a nutty, creamy, cheesy flavor, and it's a great source of B vitamins, folic acid, selenium, zinc, and even protein—which is why you'll find it in a lot of vegan recipes. The next time you make scrambled eggs, try sprinkling a little of it into the mix (I know, not vegan, but yummy).

For that little kick I mentioned, add a pinch of red pepper flakes or a teeny bit of chili powder.

  1 cup water
  2 tablespoons freshly squeezed lemon juice
  ¼ cup canned pimento, drained
  ⅔ cup whole raw almonds
1¼ teaspoons onion powder
  ¼ cup nutritional yeast
  2 teaspoons salt
  1 teaspoon red pepper flakes or chili powder, or more to taste (optional)

Put all the ingredients except red pepper flakes in a blender (preferably a Vitamix or other high-powered blender) and start blending on low speed. Switch to medium, then increase to high and blend for about 3 minutes. Taste and add red pepper flakes for a little more bang, if desired. Your vegan cheese sauce is definitely best served fresh, so pitch what you don't eat.

SALADS & DRESSINGS

SALADS & DRESSINGS

I'll be honest: I have to make myself eat salad. But the more salads I eat, the better I feel and the more I realize that there's more to a bowl of greens than iceberg lettuce and ranch dressing. Although . . . I do enjoy iceberg lettuce and ranch dressing.

Nutrition experts can't stop telling us how important dark leafy greens are, and with good reason. They have a ridiculous amount of vitamins and minerals, and the chlorophyll in these veggies keeps your colon going "Yay!" And while I used to think there was no way a salad was ever going to fill me up, I now find that adding protein (like salmon, chicken, tofu, chickpeas, or edamame), fruit (such as pears, sliced oranges, strawberries, dried cherries), and vegetables (including carrots, colorful bell peppers, beets, cherry tomatoes) to it really does the trick.

I'm also a big fan of DIY salad dressing. Good dressing makes me much more likely to polish off my salad. I love to look for local olive oils and vinegars, which gives me another good excuse to get my salad act together. (I recently went to Ojai, where I found my favorite olive oil ever; it's infused with peppers and garlic. You can actually see whole peppers and garlic in it! The only problem is that you smell rank after you eat it—Michael says he can literally smell me from across the room after I toss my lettuce or spinach in it, but he loves me anyway. I say it's worth the stink.)

Check out these recipes. They prove, once and for all, that there's nothing boring or skimpy about salad.

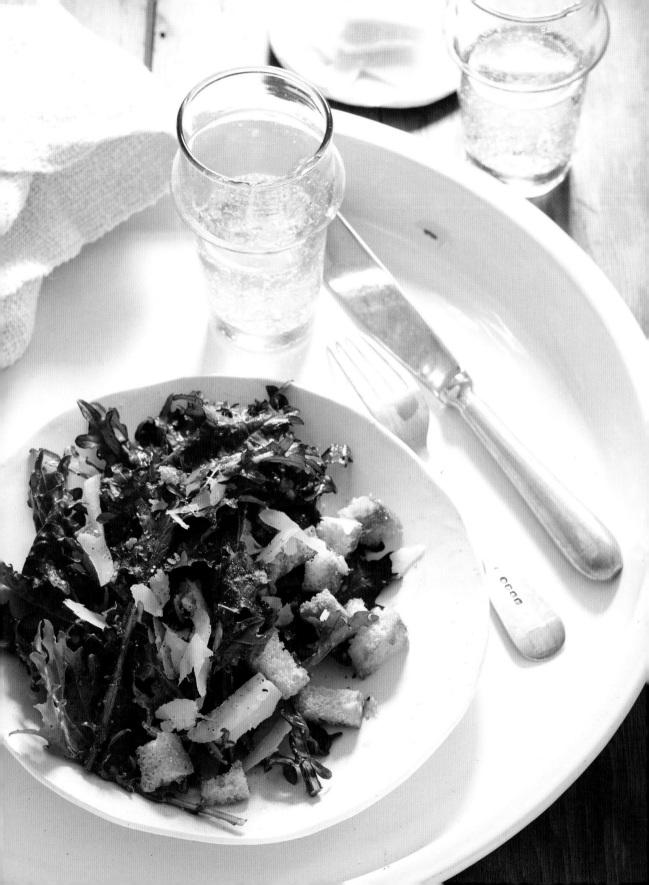

TUSCAN KALE CAESAR SALAD

Makes 4 large servings

This is a recipe my friend Christina Hendricks shared with Rachael Ray when she was on Rachael's show. You know Christina—she played the powerful role of Joan Holloway on *Mad Men*. She's just as amazing in real life as she is onscreen, and she makes one hell of a salad. The Caesar dressing is super unique because it doesn't require olive oil. Christina says that was purely accidental—she was making the recipe one day and forgot to add it. (See, even experts make mistakes sometimes!) She found that the dressing was rich and thick enough without it. But as far as oils go, olive oil is one of the best (it reduces the risk of type 2 diabetes and some cancers, and it's very good for your heart), so feel free to add 2 to 3 tablespoons to this recipe if you have a hankering for it.

Don't be daunted by the eggs. You're going to boil some water and dip two eggs into the boiling water for about 45 seconds so they're a little warmed through. Then you'll crack them open and use one whole egg (white and yolk), plus just the yolk of the other, to make the dressing.

Whenever I make this, I make a ton because it's so delicious and keeps well in the fridge.

  3 tablespoons freshly squeezed lemon juice
1½ teaspoons anchovy paste
  ½ cup grated Parmesan cheese, plus more for serving (optional)
  3 garlic cloves, minced
  1 whole egg and 1 yolk, boiled for 45 seconds (see headnote)
Dash of Worcestershire sauce
Freshly ground black pepper, to taste
  2 heads black Tuscan kale, regular kale, or romaine
Garlic croutons, for serving (optional)

Mix the lemon juice, anchovy paste, Parmesan, garlic, whole egg and yolk, Worcestershire, and pepper in a medium bowl. Clean the kale, remove the stems, pat it dry, and tear it into bite-size pieces. Add the kale to a large bowl, pour the dressing over the kale, and toss to coat. If you'd like, you can top the salad with a little more Parmesan and some homemade garlic croutons.

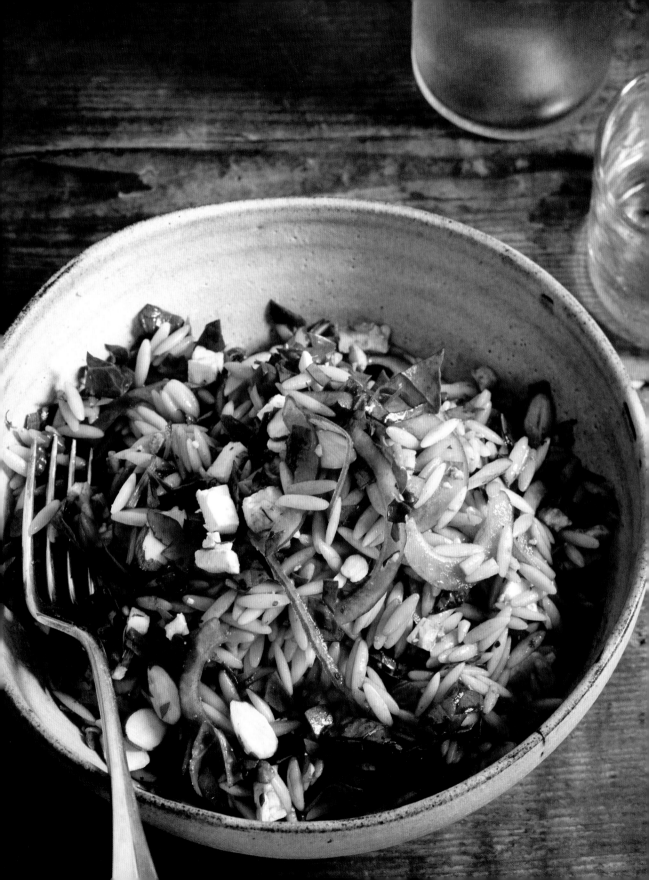

SPINACH SALAD WITH ORZO

Makes 6 to 8 servings

I'm a spinach monster, and I'm all over this spinach salad. Spinach is a very good alternative when you're starting to burn out on mesclun or kale salads. And it's one of the healthiest foods ever, packed with vitamins that (yes, Popeye) boost your bones and fight colds. Spinach is known to have anti-inflammatory and anti-cancer benefits as well. It has a slightly sweet flavor, which is why a lot of people like to add something sweet to a spinach salad, like strawberries or poppy seed dressing, which is always delish. But by adding a little pasta to your salad—along with salty feta, zesty red onion, and subtly sweet almonds—you end up with something hearty, filling, *and* flavorful. (You can skip the almonds if you're not a nut nut.)

1 (16-ounce) package orzo pasta
1 (10-ounce) package baby spinach leaves, finely chopped
½ pound crumbled feta cheese (1 cup)
½ red onion, finely chopped
¾ cup sliced almonds
½ teaspoon dried basil
¼ teaspoon freshly ground white pepper
½ cup olive oil
½ cup balsamic vinegar

Bring a large pot of water to a boil and cook the orzo according to the package instructions or to your liking. (I prefer it al dente, or a little bit firm.) Drain, rinse, and refrigerate it until it's cool enough not to wilt your spinach.

Mix the spinach with the feta, onion, almonds, basil, and white pepper in a large bowl. Toss with the orzo and finish with the oil and vinegar.

CHICKPEA SALAD WITH DRIED CHERRIES

Makes 4 servings

This is a perfectly balanced salad, with its fresh, slightly bitter greens, protein-packed chickpeas, and sweet dried cherries. I like to make it with a little balsamic dressing (like my Basic Balsamic Vinaigrette, page 85) to get a burst of different flavors in my mouth. You can go light on the dill or skip it altogether if you're not a fan.

- 6 cups mesclun mix
- 2 carrots, thinly sliced lengthwise
- 1 (15-ounce) can chickpeas, drained and rinsed
- ½ cup dried cherries, cranberries, or golden raisins
- ¼ cup fresh dill sprigs
- Dressing of your choice

Toss all the ingredients with dressing and enjoy!

BASIC BALSAMIC VINAIGRETTE

Makes about ¾ cup, enough for a family-size salad

There are a million ways to make a balsamic vinaigrette, but this is one of my favorites. Classic, tangy, and fresh, this dressing goes well with just about any salad, especially ones with sweet elements like cheese or fruit. And if you want to sweeten this dressing up, you can add a teaspoon of honey.

3 tablespoons balsamic vinegar
1 tablespoon Dijon mustard
1 garlic clove, minced
1 teaspoon honey (optional)
½ cup olive oil
Salt and freshly ground black pepper, to taste
Lemon juice, to taste

Mix the vinegar, Dijon, garlic, and honey, if using, in a bowl. Pour the oil in slowly, whisking to mix it completely. Add salt and pepper to taste. Add a squeeze of lemon to taste. Store the dressing in a glass bottle or jar in your fridge; it will last for several weeks. Give it a shake before using.

MICHAEL'S HEALTHY FRESH
SALAD DRESSING

Makes 2 servings

I learned this one from Michael, who has been making this dressing forever. It has very complex flavors—tart, sweet, and tangy—all rolled into one easy-to-make dressing. We toss it with a bright summer salad or just some baby arugula and serve it whenever we have guests.

     Juice of 1 large lemon
 ½ teaspoon Dijon mustard
 ½ teaspoon honey
     Pinch or two of finely chopped fresh parsley
 ¾ teaspoon salt
 ½ teaspoon freshly ground black pepper
 1 small garlic clove, finely chopped

Whisk everything together in a bowl, or throw all the ingredients in a small sealed jar or other container and shake it like a Polaroid picture!

BETH'S FIELD GUIDE TO COMMON GREENS

As a greens-eating novice, I didn't know my radicchio from my romaine. Half the time I wasn't sure if I was supposed to eat these greens or put them in a vase with water. But I've done some experimentation and some research, and I finally feel like I'm a mean greens-eating machine. Hopefully this section will help guide you through the produce aisle and turn you into a greens goddess. And it's always good to buy this stuff at the farmers' market when you can.

Just remember: Green is great—green vegetables, green fruit, eating things that come from our green Earth—until one day, it isn't, and you just have to eat a peanut butter and jelly sandwich and that's that. Fine, fantastic. Enjoy it, then get back to green the next day.

Arugula
Eruca sativa

Okay, turns out that arugula is not a lettuce (which is what I always thought), but an edible vegetable rich in vitamins A and C and potassium. It's a tiny bit bitter, a tiny bit sweet, and a tiny bit peppery. Give it a whiff and you'll recognize its distinctive scent. Try mixing it into your salads with other greens or sprinkling a bit on your pizza for pizzazz. It tastes soooo good with tomatoes and cheese! But eat it quickly—it will only stay fresh in your refrigerator for a couple of days.

Cabbage (red, green, savoy)
Brassicaceae

Cabbage is not a lettuce either—it is a cruciferous vegetable like kale and broccoli. But you can still chop it up and throw it in your salads and give it the lettuce treatment. The cabbage won't fight back. Health experts go nuts about the benefits of cabbage consumption—it's full of antioxidants! It's anti-inflammatory and can help prevent cancer! It's also been studied for its assistance in relieving stomach ailments and cardiovascular issues. What it

legendarily will not relieve is GAS—too much cabbage and you'll be able to
shoot yourself out of your kitchen on fumes alone! Wash it as you use it and
wrap the rest in plastic and store it in your fridge; it could last you months.

Chard
Beta vulgaris subsp. vulgaris

Swiss chard stands out in the produce aisle: It looks tall and regal, with
elegant leaves and crunchy stalks that are white, red, or yellow. You'll find
this vegetable in a lot of Mediterranean dishes, and it's no wonder why: Chard
is filled with nutrients and antioxidants that would make other vegetables
green with jealousy if they weren't green already—even chard's close relations,
beets and spinach. Store it unwashed in your fridge, and it will last for two to
three days.

Collard greens
Brassica oleracea

Southern cooks love collard greens! And with good reason—they're full of
vitamins and a wonderful source of calcium and antioxidants that are
rumored to lower risk of heart disease and cancer. Cabbage, a cousin of collard
greens, is like, "Whatever, you're the greatest, fine." Rinse collard greens
well before you trim the stalks and cook the dark-green leaves, which have
a hearty, meaty goodness. Keep them refrigerated and wrapped in plastic to
retain moisture, and get rid of greens if they turn yellow or stinky. They
should last for a couple of weeks.

Cress (garden)
Lepidium sativum

Turns out cress is an herb! Its tops burst with tangy, peppery joy, which is
just as tasty on sandwiches as it is sprinkled over soups or salads (try it in
place of sprouts). Rinse your cress, trim the stems, then blot with a paper towel.
Refrigerate in a plastic bag and use within four to five days.

Endive (Belgian)
Cichorium endivia

Finally, an answer on the great endive-pronunciation debate: You give its name a Belgian phonetic twist and call it "on-deev," as opposed to "en-dive." En garde! Add this lightly bitter chicory to your salads for a boost of potassium and fiber, or consider replacing a cracker with a nice firm leaf of endive. Wash it as you use it and store the rest in a plastic bag in the refrigerator for four to five days, or until the leaves begin to brown/wilt.

Escarole
Cichorium endivia

A fellow chicory, escarole has a faintly bitter flavor. Its leaves are curly and wild . . . sending poor plain lettuce back to the refrigerator bin with a sigh of jealousy. And what a zesty twist it gives to soups! Of course it is full of vitamins, especially folic acid, which is so good for mothers-to-be. Eat the tender, light-green inner leaves raw or add them to fruit salads, and throw the tougher, darker leaves into recipes. Wash by filling a bowl with cold water, adding your escarole, and swirling the leaves around until any dirt falls to the bottom of the bowl. Pat dry and keep in a plastic bag in the fridge for two to three weeks.

Kale
Brassica oleracea

Kale, kale, the superhero, the superfood! It's more than a trend . . . more than a moment . . . kale is on everyone's lips, quite literally. Kale is antioxidant, anti-inflammatory, cholesterol-lowering, cardiovascular-benefiting, and rumored to have cancer-preventative benefits . . . plus it has a taste that keeps you wanting more (one of my friends loves it because it's so fulfilling to chew, chew, chew). Though it looks lettuce-like, it's actually a descendant of the wild cabbage, making it a closer relation to broccoli and cauliflower than a head of iceberg. You can eat it raw in salads . . . on a burger . . . or steam it to your heart's content. Wash it as you use it and keep the rest in a plastic bag in the fridge for up to five days.

LETTUCES
Lactuca sativa

Butter/Boston/Bibb

All three of these are considered "butterhead" lettuces, but Bibb is a little bit smaller. These varieties are appreciated for their smooth and tender leaves and sweet flavor (at least as far as lettuce goes). They are full of essential nutrients and vitamins, particularly A, C, and K. Toss them with your favorite toppings (their leaves hold dressing so nicely), add them to sandwiches, or use them as wraps. The three Bs usually cost a bit more than other lettuces, but hey, you may enjoy them more! Store unwashed and give them a good rinse with cold water when you're ready to use them.

Iceberg

Poor iceberg (also known as "crisphead"). Dark-leafy-green enthusiasts just stomp on its head. But fear not—even if you're eating iceberg salads, you're not totally missing out on nutrition. It, too, has nutrients, along with much more water than other lettuces, making it hydrating. It also tends to be a bit less pricey. Just avoid the temptation of regularly eating an iceberg wedge salad with blue cheese and bacon—that's basically using your lettuce as a delivery system for delicious but not exactly heart-healthy fats (which I think are fine in moderation)! Fun fact: There is no ice in iceberg lettuce— its name comes from the fact that it was transported on ice in the 1920s. Tear the leaves by hand to avoid browning, and keep in a plastic bag in your fridge for up to a week.

Leaf (green, red)

Not all lettuce comes from a head, as you may have noticed at your local salad bar. Leaves that branch from a single stalk are called leaf lettuces, and they tend to have a little more flavor than the average head. Sadly, they don't last quite as long in your fridge, but you'd be surprised by how quickly you'll go through them. You can buy them prewashed, but if they're not, wash the leaves, blot with paper towels, and store in your fridge for up to three days.

Mustard greens
Brassica juncea

People from around the world have been eating mustard greens for over five thousand years, enjoying their antioxidant and anti-inflammatory benefits. These little guys can lower bad cholesterol and possibly ward off cancer. You can eat them raw or sauté them. Wrap unwashed mustard greens in paper towel and keep them in a high-humidity storage drawer in the fridge for up to five days.

Parsley
Petroselinum crispum

Parsley is actually an herb, but you should eat it like it's a veg because it's so darn good for you. It's a great source of minerals and antioxidant vitamins, so don't be dissing parsley as a lowly garnish when it can be so much more. You can use it in vegetable dishes, as well as chicken, fish, and meat dishes—and don't forget to add it to your salsa verde. Ay caramba! You can store it unwashed at room temperature or in the fridge; it should stay fresh for up to three weeks.

Radicchio
Cichorium intybus

Commonly thought by many of my drama school classmates to be a lower character in Shakespeare's canon, radicchio is actually a superfood that can look like a small head of cabbage or the aforementioned endive, just red in color. Also known as "Italian chicory," it is delicious paired with arugula and, ahem, pear. See what I did there? Pair . . . pear. Balsamic vinaigrette and honey, we're coming! Store unwashed radicchio in a plastic bag in the refrigerator for two to three weeks.

Romaine (a.k.a. cos)

Romaine was first grown in the Papal gardens of Rome, ergo the name "romaine." It's a nice, fibrous leaf with relatively mild flavor and an excellent source of vitamin C, folic acid, and potassium. The stalks tend to be longer and straighter than the round heads of iceberg or butter lettuce. Wash and dry it before storing in a plastic bag in the fridge; it will last you about five days. While this is the lettuce you'll find in most Caesar salads, feel free to also add it to a smoothie! Hail Caesar! PS: Cut off the tips at the top, as they tend to have a bitter taste.

Spinach
Spinacia oleracea

The vitamins . . . the minerals . . . the dietary fiber! Chenopods like beets, chard, quinoa, and spinach are irresistible for their combination of good taste + being good for you. Raw or lightly cooked, spinach is an ideal addition to salads, sides, and smoothies. Remember that spinach shrinks quite a bit as you cook it, so don't be stingy with your portions. And this is just a personal opinion, but I believe that where there's spinach, garlic should never be far behind (except when making smoothies, of course)! Store loosely packed in a plastic bag in your refrigerator crisper, and it should last four to five days.

Watercress
Nasturtium officinale

That tiny, crisp member of the mustard family you find in your soup or salad is watercress, an herb that's been considered a healer since, like, Olden Times. Hippocrates used fresh watercress to treat patients, and in the 1700s people believed that watercress could cleanse the blood. It has more iron than spinach, more calcium than milk, and more vitamin C than oranges. So don't wait for high tea—add watercress to everything today! Submerge the stems in water, pat them dry, loosely cover the leaves in plastic or in a slightly opened plastic bag, and store in the fridge. Just use it quickly—magical watercress only stays fresh for a couple of days.

SIDES

Sides are my favorite part of a meal. Frankly, I think it's side-ist that sides are called "sides," when if it were up to me they'd be front and center in a meal. Fine, I'll say it: It's okay if once in a while your meal is just sweet potato fries and curried cauliflower. See you next time, Entrée!

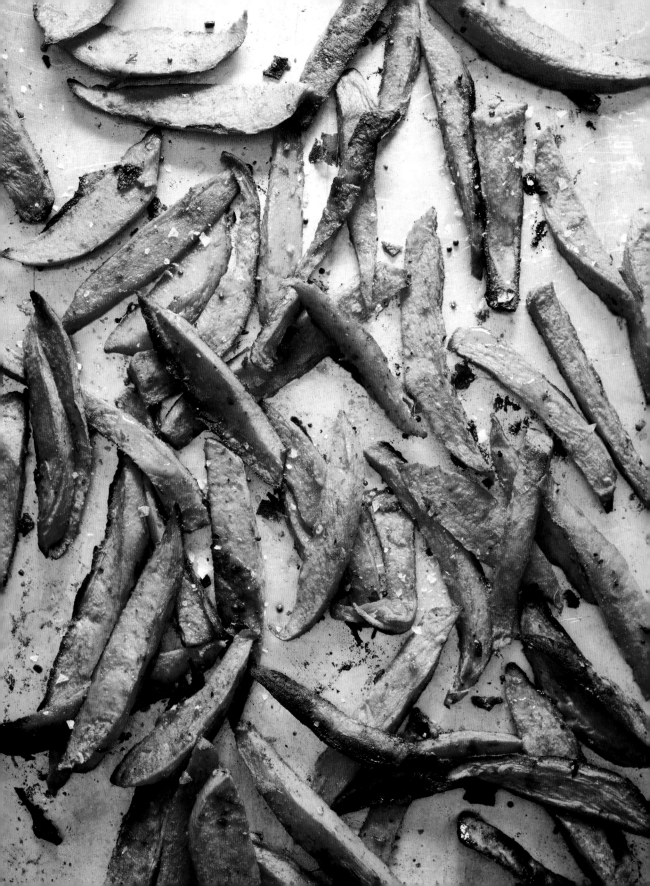

BAKED SWEET POTATO FRIES

Makes 2 to 4 servings

If you're in the mood for a quick and yummy meal or you're making something super healthy like chicken or salmon and need a little va-va-voom on the side, these fries will do the trick. Crunchy on the outside and creamy on the inside, with a little bit of sweetness, they're the ultimate in healthy comfort food. They're good for entertaining, feeding picky eaters, or when you need a starchy food without any guilt. And sweet potatoes are packed with beta-carotene, which is good for your vision, immunity, and overall health; and vitamin A, which supports healthy skin, teeth, and bones.

But what makes this recipe the most fun is that you can add your own spice rub to the potatoes. I've never made a batch that didn't work.

   2 pounds sweet potatoes (about 3 large)
   ¼ cup olive oil (use 2 tablespoons if you're cutting down on fat)
   1 tablespoon sugar
   1 tablespoon salt
   1 to 2 tablespoons spice or combination of spices (chipotle powder, smoked paprika, Chinese 5-spice powder, pumpkin pie spice, garam masala, Cajun seasoning)
Nonstick cooking spray (optional)

Preheat the oven to 450°F. (For crispier fries, preheat the oven to 500°F.)

Peel the sweet potatoes and trim off the ends. Cut the potatoes in half lengthwise, then in half crosswise. Cut each piece into wedges. (I prefer mine thin, the width of traditional french fries; Michael prefers his thick, the width of steak fries.)

Put the sweet potatoes in a large bowl, add the olive oil, and mix well. Sprinkle the potatoes with the sugar, salt, and spice(s) of your choice. Mix with your hands and make sure all the pieces are well coated.

Spread the sweet potatoes in a single layer on a baking sheet. (The oil they are coated with should keep them from sticking to the pan, so no need to oil or line the baking sheet. If you reduced the amount of oil, spray the baking sheet with nonstick cooking spray or line with parchment.)

Bake for 15 minutes, then remove the baking sheet from the oven and turn over all the sweet potato pieces. Return the pan to the oven and bake for another 10 to 15 minutes, or until the potatoes are well browned and tender. Let them cool for 5 minutes before serving.

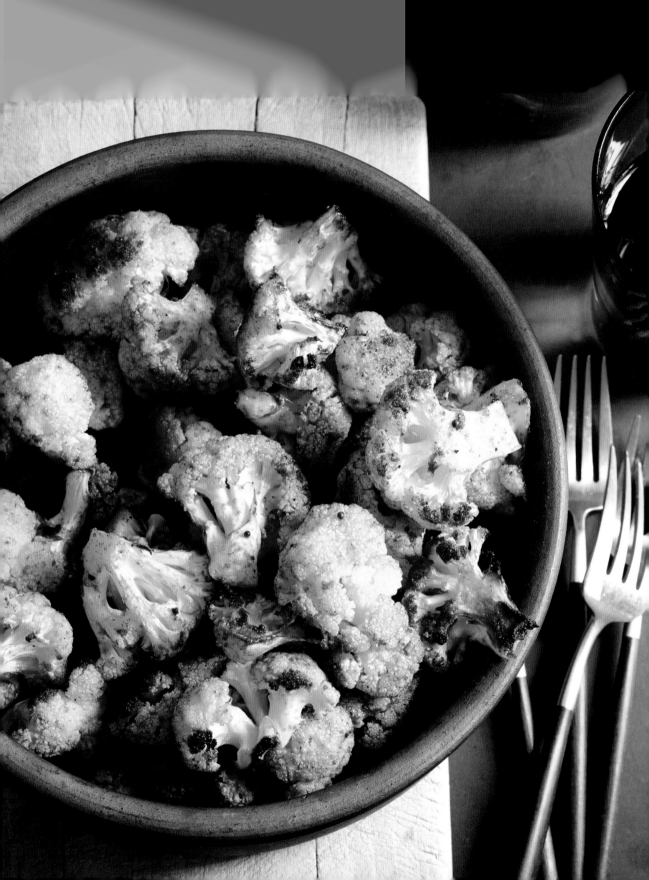

GRAMMY'S CURRIED CAULIFLOWER

Makes 4 servings

If you'd asked me to try curry powder as a kid, I would have been like, "Ewww, gross!" But today, curry is one of my favorite spice blends. Cauliflower + curry? Fuggedaboutit. Who would have thought that cauliflower could be so delish? Not my extended family—they had never eaten cauliflower before I made this recipe for them, BUT THEY LOVED IT. Grammy got a taste of India! She loved it, and you will, too. Cauliflower is beloved by nutrition experts for its anti-inflammatory and antioxidant qualities. And it has an almost sweet and creamy flavor, making it satisfying in an unexpected way, especially as a great potato substitute.

1 head cauliflower, cut into bite-size pieces (about 4 cups)
2 tablespoons coconut oil, melted
1 tablespoon freshly squeezed lemon juice
1 tablespoon curry powder
¼ teaspoon salt

Preheat the oven to 450°F.

Put all the ingredients in a big bowl and toss to coat the cauliflower evenly.

Spread the cauliflower in a single layer on a baking sheet and bake for 20 minutes, or until golden and tender.

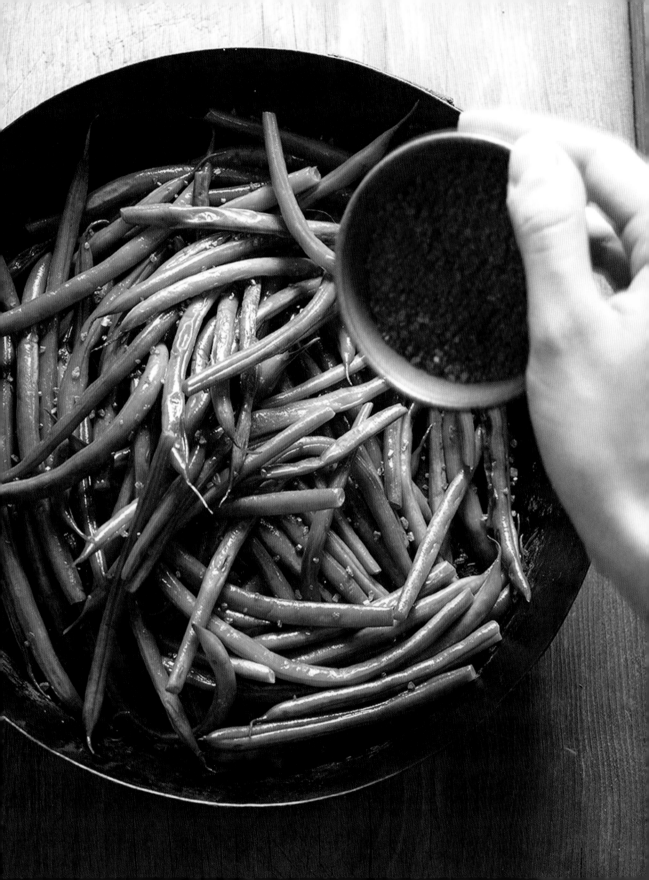

GREEN BEANS WITH FLAVA

Makes 2 servings

This is a fast and easy side dish that goes well with traditional "American" dishes like chicken, turkey, and red meat, but also with Asian- and Indian-style entrées. It's also a great snack. When that french-fry feeling comes on, like you want to keep picking up something and putting it in your mouth, try making these instead—it'll take you less than ten minutes.

 1 pound fresh green beans
 Olive oil, about a 3-second pour
 Flavored salt, freshly ground black pepper,
     and/or red pepper flakes, to taste

Bring a pot of water to a boil and boil the green beans for about 4 minutes. Drain the beans, pat dry, and put them in a skillet over low heat. Add the olive oil and shake the pan a bit to coat the beans. They will start to crisp within a couple of minutes; keep your heat low enough so that they don't burn. Once crisp, remove from the heat and sprinkle them with flavored salt, black pepper, and/or pepper flakes. Himalayan sea salt gives these excellent flavor.

> If you like your green beans crunchier, skip the boiling step and simply pan-fry them for a few extra minutes.

SAVORY ROASTED POTATOES & SPROUTS

Makes 3 to 4 servings

When you're cooking with rosemary, you can't *not* get excited to eat. It's one of my favorite herbs to grow in my garden, and I find the smell so yummy and calming. Also, I love fingerling potatoes—and not just for dinner but brunch, too. Along with Brussels sprouts, they make a cool combo—so thanks to Oh She Glows for putting them together in this recipe, which I've tweaked to my taste. I don't know why Brussels sprouts got such a lousy reputation; roast them until they're caramelized and crispy, and they're pop-in-your-mouth good. When you combine the dense texture of the Brussels sprouts with the creaminess of the potatoes, it's kind of like Thanksgiving in your mouth. And that line right there is why I'm not a food writer.

1¾ pounds fingerling potatoes
¾ pound Brussels sprouts
3 garlic cloves, minced
2 tablespoons minced fresh rosemary
1 tablespoon plus 1 teaspoon extra-virgin olive oil
¾ teaspoon kosher salt, or more to taste
Freshly ground black pepper, to taste
¼ teaspoon red pepper flakes (optional)

Preheat the oven to 400°F and line a large baking sheet with parchment paper.

Rinse the potatoes and pat them dry. Leave the potatoes unpeeled and slice them in half lengthwise; add them to a large mixing bowl.

Trim the stems off the Brussels sprouts and remove any loose outer leaves. Add them to the bowl with the potatoes.

Add the garlic, rosemary, and oil to the bowl, along with a sprinkle of salt, pepper, and red pepper flakes, if using. Toss with your hands to combine and spread the mixture in a single layer on the baking sheet.

Roast for 35 to 38 minutes, stirring halfway through, until the potatoes are golden and the sprouts are lightly charred. Season with salt and pepper to taste and serve pronto.

PALEO BREAD

Makes 1 loaf

This is based on a recipe for the Paleo bread from Elana's Pantry. Elana Amsterdam suffered from celiac disease and eventually switched to a Paleo diet, going totally grain-free. The whole idea of the Paleo diet is a "whole" idea—you try to eat whole foods that mimic what our ancestors ate back in Paleolithic, hunter-gatherer times. This does not necessarily mean Fred Flintstone chowing down on a bronto burger . . . well, at least not the bun. Paleo is high-protein, low-carb, high-fiber eating, with almost zero allowance for processed foods. While I can't follow these guidelines full-time, I can definitely sign off on the game plan—and it's a sound strategy for gluten-free eaters. If you want to try it out, Elena's recipes are terrific, tasty, and so good for you (elanaspantry.com). I like this bread as a snack—especially before a workout because it gives you a burst of healthy-carbohydrate energy—and it's great for breakfast.

     2 cups blanched almond flour
     2 tablespoons coconut flour
     ¼ cup golden flaxmeal
     ¼ teaspoon kosher salt
     ½ teaspoon baking soda
     5 large eggs, room temperature
     1 tablespoon coconut oil
     1 tablespoon honey
     1 tablespoon cider vinegar

Preheat the oven to 350°F and grease a 7½ x 3½-inch loaf pan.

Place the almond flour, coconut flour, flaxmeal, salt, and baking soda in a blender and pulse the ingredients together. Then pulse in the eggs, oil, honey, and vinegar until well combined.

Transfer the batter to the greased pan and bake for 30 minutes, or until it's a little brown on top.

Let cool in the pan and then serve. This will keep in your refrigerator for 5 to 6 days.

ASK A NUTRITIONIST

After thinking about food so much, I had a bunch of nutrition questions. And so did many of you when I asked you to send them my way on social media. I passed them on to registered dietician Michelle Allison, a.k.a. The Fat Nutritionist, and asked for her advice.

If I'm eating healthfully, do I still need to take a multivitamin?
Not necessarily, though there are times when vitamin supplementation is useful. If you eat enough food, and get enough variety, most people will get their needs met just fine. Older adults, especially those living at higher latitudes where there is less sunlight throughout the year, may need additional vitamin D. You can get blood-work done through your doctor if you're worried about a particular deficiency.

It's not a good idea to get more than the Tolerable Upper Limit (UL) of vitamins and minerals, as it can actually increase risk of certain health problems. You can look up the UL for all vitamins and minerals by Googling the Dietary Reference Intakes (DRIs.)

If I don't eat much dairy, where can I add calcium to my diet? Is soy milk bad for me?
You can definitely get calcium without dairy. Here are some nondairy calcium sources:

- soy yogurt, fortified soy beverages, and other fortified nondairy beverages like rice and almond drinks
- soybeans, navy beans, white beans, and tofu prepared with calcium sulfate
- almonds
- sesame seed paste (tahini)
- blackstrap molasses
- some vegetables, such as bok choy, okra, collard greens, and turnip greens
- some fruit, like figs and fortified orange juice

No, soy milk is not bad for you. Particularly, fortified soy beverages with at least 7 grams of protein per serving can be a crucial part of the diet, especially if you're avoiding animal products. Regarding soy and health, particularly breast-cancer risk, the research is ongoing, but at present there isn't any evidence to suggest that eating about 2 servings of soy foods per day increases health risks. Some people report having more GI symptoms and menstrual symptoms if they consume soy, but this is probably individual. If you tolerate soy well, there's no special reason not to eat it.

If you have hypothyroidism, you may want to talk to your doctor if you rely a lot on soy-based foods or supplements because your thyroid-replacement medication dose may need adjustment.

Is it worth spending extra $ on organic food? If so, what should I spend it on (Organic fruit? Veggies? Meat?)
This is really a personal choice, and there are a lot of arguments on both sides of this issue—health arguments as well as political ones. If you have trouble affording food in general, paying extra for organic is probably not worth it. For most people, getting more fruits and vegetables, conventional OR organic, is healthier than worrying too much about how they were grown.

If you like organic produce more, or it aligns with your values and politics more, AND you can afford it, buy it and enjoy it. If it doesn't make a difference to you, buy conventional and don't stress. There are compelling arguments to be made about the environmental impact of both conventionally grown and organic produce. Both are fine choices.

I love sweets. Is it better to eat a little bit of the real thing or a lot of the "diet" version (for example, real ice cream vs. frozen yogurt)?
It's better to eat what you truly like. Sometimes I actually like the "diet" version more, though usually I prefer nondiet versions—but you never know. Try things and make a decision based on what your taste buds and body tell you. In my opinion, it's better to be truly satisfied by what you eat. If you feel that something isn't satisfying, you're going to go looking for more, or for something else that is. Just eat what you truly want from the start and skip the drama. If you're worried about nutrition, combine the food you're craving with a meal or well-rounded snack and pat yourself on the back for being a grown-up about it.

What are "inflammatory" foods, and what exactly do they inflame?
Inflammation usually refers to something that triggers an immune response in the body. Sometimes people get an inflammatory response to certain foods because

they have a food allergy, or sometimes because they have an autoimmune disease (like celiac disease or inflammatory bowel disease) that causes inflammation. A lot of diseases involve an inflammatory component. It's obvious when you've got the flu and your throat is swelled up and your nose is running, but inflammation is a part of chronic diseases like cardiovascular disease, too, just not as obvious.

Eating a healthy diet can help reduce chronic inflammation, and thereby reduce chronic-disease risk, and there is some ongoing research about the effects of a Mediterranean diet (for example) on inflammation in the body, and specific types of oils and plant chemicals on inflammation. There is also a book about inflammatory foods that contains a rating system (based on several factors) that lists which foods are more inflammatory and which are less. This might be helpful to some people; however, the author cautions that several otherwise-healthy foods have an inflammatory rating, and that this does not mean you should stop eating them. Even within the context of the anti-inflammatory diet she promotes, she encourages getting a mix of different foods and overall balance. That is good nutrition advice for anyone.

For people who are still trying to get down the basics of healthy eating (like having regular meals, understanding hunger and fullness, and getting enough fruits and veggies), taking inflammation into account might be too complicated and stress-inducing. Focus on eating foods you enjoy, notice your hunger and fullness cues, and add on any missing food groups, first and foremost. Then, if you feel like complicating things further, go for it. If doing so makes you regress, stop and stick with the basics.

What are some sneaky ways to get more veggies into my meals?
Making vegetables in an enjoyable way is much better than trying to sneak anything or trick yourself. But most sauces are easy to add veggies to—for example, extra chopped-up onions or celery or green peppers go well in tomato-based spaghetti sauce. But if you really think you don't like vegetables and you feel obligated to eat them, why not try to see if a different way of preparing them improves things? Most vegetables that taste awful when boiled to death, or when steamed with nothing added, are actually really tasty when drizzled with olive oil, tossed with garlic, and roasted on a baking sheet in the oven for 20 minutes. Most vegetables are better (and your vitamin absorption is better) when you put fat on them—could be oil, cheese, butter. Eating a vegetable is better than not eating a vegetable, even if you're dipping it in ranch.

Try making them tasty first. Then notice how you feel on days you eat them vs. days when you don't. If they taste good and you feel good when you eat them, you'll want to eat them. No sneaking required.

What is your go-to healthy snack?
Anything that contains protein, carbs, and fat (and usually a fruit or vegetable) works for me. Sometimes that's cheese and crackers, or carrots and hummus, or a cookie with nuts and an apple. An apple even makes peanut M&M's stick around longer.

Is the whole "gluten-free" thing a trend, or is it here to stay?
It's not a trend for people with celiac disease! For everyone else—for people who truly do not experience any kind of symptoms of intolerance, allergy, or autoimmune disease with gluten—I'm pretty sure it's a fad. There is a long and colorful history of diet fads going back to the nineteenth century, and if you've been around long enough to see some of them come and go, or if you've read the history, it becomes pretty clear which ones are fads. But fads usually come back around, slightly repackaged. So gluten-free for people who don't actually have a reason to be gluten-free will probably come back around, in a slightly different form, at some point. It will cycle in and out of fashion.

What's my best option to eat in a fast-food joint?
I just try to find something that includes a vegetable, which usually means adding a salad on the side. Take into account how hungry you are and order accordingly. Some days will be hungry value-meal days. Other days you will be less hungry, but if you're in the habit of ordering the value meal, it will still be tempting. If you're truly less hungry, you can try experimenting with a smaller item—it might be something à la carte, or off the kids' menu, or a salad.

I love cereal. What's my best choice?
What leaves you feeling nourished? What leaves you satisfied?
For me, the answer is Frosted Mini-Wheats. For you, it might be something else. Pay attention and your body will let you know. (*Note from Beth to reader: Just take it easy on the Froot Loops!*)

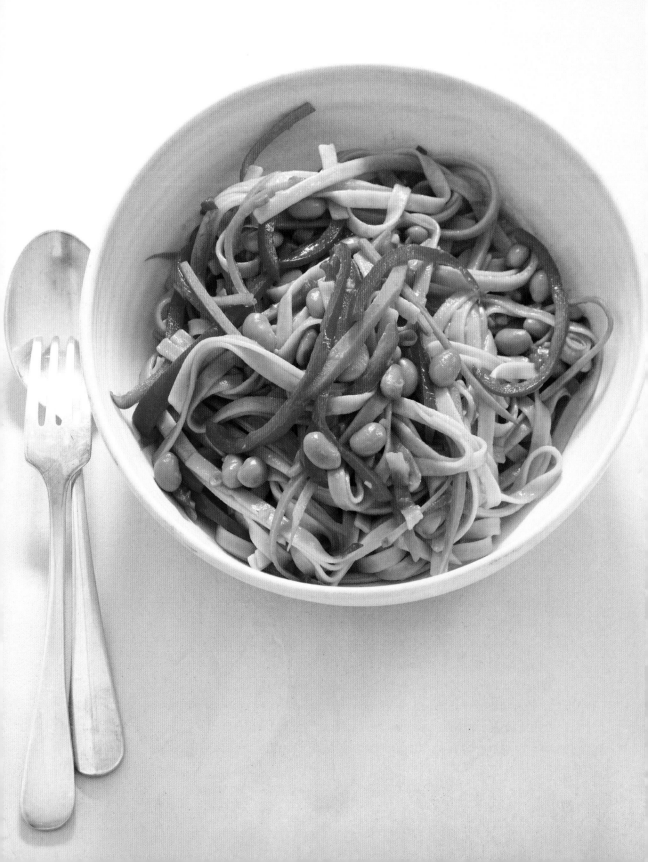

CHAPTER 5

MAXIMIZE MEALS:
MAIN DISHES

You've got the food, you've got the equipment, you've got the practice under your belt (which may be getting looser). Now it's time to make an entrée into cooking entrées. The recipes that follow are delicious, fun to make, cost-conscious, and good for your bod. So take a look around your kitchen. Give a friendly wave to your blender, your mixing bowls, your roasting pan . . . these are now nice, familiar friends. 'Cause it's time to (game show music here) MAXIMIZE MEALS! It's the next step in your kitchen-comfort evolution. You now know why we're eating so many of the foods in this book—so let's start making them, meal-size.

MAIN DISHES

VEGAN LO MEIN

Makes 4 servings

I was devastated when my roommates Alisha and Courtney became vegan. (They read *Skinny Bitch*, and that was that.) How could they do this to me? They were my doughnut- and egg-eating buddies (though, not at the same time). Even though I knew Courtney was an amazing cook, I was certain that I wasn't going to like anything she made that was vegan. Then she made me this lo mein recipe with edamame, or shelled soybeans, and I was like, "Girls' night again next weekend?!"

I love to eat a plant-based diet, but I can't do a 100 percent vegan. I've watched a ton of documentaries, and I know that many people feel that a vegan diet is the healthiest way to go . . . but I could barely get through my workweek without eating some animal protein (and good carbs). Protein builds muscle mass, which is helpful to me when I'm trying to remember all my lines and prancing around in stilettos all day.

Everybody's body is different, and you have to listen to yours.

That said, I make this dish to eat on show night because it gives me lots of fuel (protein from the soybeans, plus carbohydrates from the quinoa or pasta), and it's filling in a good way (not a gross, bloated way). I know there's a little sugar in this recipe, which isn't a crime, but you can skip it and still get great flavor. It does take a little time to make, so open a bottle of wine and enjoy the process.

    8 to 10 ounces whole wheat or brown rice pasta,
       or 1 to 1¼ cups quinoa
    2 cups frozen edamame
    ¼ cup vegetable stock
    ¼ cup rice vinegar
    3 tablespoons soy sauce
    2 teaspoons raw sugar
    2 teaspoons toasted sesame oil
    ⅛ teaspoon red pepper flakes
    4 scallions, thinly sliced (green part only)
    3 tablespoons olive oil, divided
    2 to 4 garlic cloves (depending on how much you like garlic), minced
    2 medium carrots, cut into matchsticks
    2 small red bell peppers, cored, seeded, and cut into matchsticks
    1 to 2 red jalapeño peppers (depending on their
       spice level and your love of spice), finely chopped

continues

continued

Bring a large pot of water to a boil. Add the pasta or quinoa and edamame and cook, stirring occasionally, until the pasta is just tender (8 to 10 minutes, or follow the package directions) or the quinoa is cooked. Drain the pasta.

Meanwhile, mix the stock, vinegar, soy sauce, sugar, sesame oil, and red pepper flakes in a small bowl until the sugar is dissolved. Stir in the scallions.

Heat 2 tablespoons of the olive oil in a large, nonstick skillet over high heat. Add the garlic and cook until just fragrant, about 30 seconds. Add the carrots, bell peppers, and jalapeños and cook, stirring often, until they are slightly softened, 3 to 4 minutes. Remove the vegetables and add the remaining tablespoon of olive oil to the pan, followed by the pasta or quinoa and edamame. Cook, stirring occasionally, until the pasta or quinoa is crispy in spots, 1 to 2 minutes. Return the cooked vegetables to the pan, add the sauce, and stir until combined. Cook until everything is warmed through and serve.

MAKE IT YOUR OWN

Try green/string beans or snow peas instead of the edamame (they're lower in protein but still delish).

SPICY INDIAN CHICKEN
& SPINACH SAAGWALA

Makes 4 servings

Michael created this recipe all on his own, and now we make it at least once a week (and it heats up great for lunch the next day). Saagwala (or "saag") is a curry dish you'll find in any Indian restaurant, with a lot of variations; chicken with spinach is a very popular combo. We call this dish our "cold buster" because the ginger, turmeric, spinach, and garlic will knock a cold right out of you. Curcumin, an active ingredient in turmeric, is an antioxidant that protects the body's cells from the damage that can become a risk factor for cancer.

BTW, we buy all of our spices fresh from our local spice shop, and we change the recipe depending on what spices we have. Sometimes we add fancy chiles, or X-tra hot fresh cayenne . . . there are no rules! (See the spice list on page 24.)

I love serving this over brown rice, but you can use basmati or jasmine if you want a sweeter, lighter flavor.

One last thought: If you're vegetarian or just not in a chicken state of mind, you can either omit the chicken or make the fragrant Red Lentils & Rice (page 115) instead.

- ¼ teaspoon ground cinnamon
- 1 teaspoon ground turmeric (add more if you're fighting a cold)
- 1 teaspoon cayenne pepper
- 2 teaspoons garam masala
- 1 teaspoon vindaloo curry powder
- 1 teaspoon ground coriander
- ¼ cup olive oil
- ½ white onion, finely chopped
- ½ teaspoon peeled and chopped fresh ginger
- 1 jalapeño pepper, finely chopped (optional)
- Salt and freshly ground black pepper, to taste
- 3 garlic cloves, finely chopped
- ½ (5-ounce) bag/tub fresh spinach (add more if you're fighting a cold!), roughly chopped
- 1 (7-ounce) container nonfat or 2% plain Greek yogurt
- ½ rotisserie chicken, skin removed, meat chopped or shredded
- 1 cup cooked brown rice

continues

continued

Toast the spices over medium-low heat in a dry pan, just until fragrant. Add the olive oil to the warm spices and cook for about a minute. Add the onion, ginger, and jalapeño, if using, and sauté until the onions soften, about 8 to 10 minutes. Add salt and pepper to taste.

Add the garlic and cook for about a minute, then stir in the spinach so it's well coated with the oil and spices. Once the spinach starts to wilt, add the yogurt and fold it in to combine. Finally, add the chicken. Stir it all together and heat for a couple of minutes until warmed through.

Serve over brown rice.

BEFORE MAKING MEALS . . .

You're doing a great job of preparing all these meals . . . now it's almost time to eat them! Here are a few things to keep in mind when you're about to dig in:

Book the time. Put your shopping, prepping, and cooking time on your calendar. Make it as important a to-do as getting to work on time.

Keep it boring. Make a shopping list *before* you shop and try to stick to it as much as you can (this is good for your well-being and your wallet). And don't go shopping on an empty stomach! That's how you end up coming home with deep-fried-who-knows-what-wings.

Mix it up. Don't get stuck eating the same stuff over and over again—you can find yourself in a nutritional and inspirational rut. Try to change it up. An easy way to get lots of variety in your veggies is to buy what's in season. That way you're getting foods that are fresh, at their most flavorful and nutritional peak, and always changing.

WHEN YOU'RE ABOUT TO BREAK BREAD . . .

Execute perfect plating. Filling up a smaller plate with more food rather than a larger plate with less food will trick your brain into feeling sated.

Give it a pretty presentation. Make that plate a pretty one—not the plate itself (though that helps), but what's on it. Make sure there's a lot of color, especially green, at every meal. And there should always be more veggies than proteins or carbs.

Make it camera-ready. To help prove to yourself that taking the time to cook is worth your effort—and to feel more satisfied by your meals—put in the extra energy to make sure that what you're eating not only *tastes* good and is good for you, but that it *looks* good before you eat it. Create an Instagram-worthy presentation even if you're just eating by yourself—no need to spend big $ on placemats, napkins, and flower arrangements. No matter what you're eating, take a sec to be thankful that delicious, healthy food made with self-love is going into your mouth.

AND IF YOU'RE EATING FOR ONE . . .

Don't lose your motivation to take good care of yourself when you're flying solo. For so many reasons, it's worth it to prepare a beautiful, healthy plate (see above) and enjoy it without standing at the kitchen counter or zoning out in front of the TV (unless you're watching *2 Broke Girls*, of course). Sit at the table with a plate in front of you and a napkin on your lap. And remember—most of these dishes are great the next day for lunch or frozen for future date nights . . . with yourself.

RED LENTILS & RICE

Makes 5 servings

Here's a delicious vegetarian alternative to Spicy Indian Chicken & Spinach Saagwala (page 111). It's warming and filling, and it packs Indian flavor without overloading you with spices.

1 tablespoon vegetable oil, such as sunflower or canola
1 cup diced onion
1 teaspoon peeled and grated fresh ginger
1 teaspoon ground coriander
1 teaspoon ground cumin
½ teaspoon ground turmeric
½ teaspoon vindaloo curry powder
½ teaspoon ground cinnamon
2 garlic cloves, minced
2 bay leaves
3 cups water
1½ cups dried red lentils, rinsed
¾ teaspoon salt
2 tablespoons unsalted butter or stick margarine

¾ cup chopped scallions (green part only)
1 tablespoon seeded and minced jalapeño pepper
½ teaspoon minced marash pepper (if you're looking for even more heat; optional)
3 tablespoons freshly squeezed lime juice
2 tablespoons minced fresh cilantro
1 teaspoon garam masala
2½ cups cooked brown basmati or brown rice, hot
5 tablespoons low-fat plain yogurt

Heat the vegetable oil in a large saucepan over medium-high heat. Add the onions and sauté for 6 minutes, or until the onions begin to brown. Add the ginger, coriander, cumin, turmeric, curry powder, cinnamon, garlic, and bay leaves and sauté for 1 minute. Add the water, lentils, and salt and bring to a boil. Cover, reduce the heat to medium-low, and simmer for 15 to 20 minutes, or until the lentils are tender. Discard the bay leaves.

Melt the butter in a small skillet over medium heat. It's time for peppers: Remember to be gentle with those jalapeños unless you want super spice! Add the scallions, jalapeño, and marash pepper, if using. Sauté for 5 minutes. Add this to the lentil mixture, then stir in the lime juice, cilantro, and garam masala.

Place ½ cup of rice into the bottom of 5 shallow bowls. Spoon about ¾ cup of the lentil mixture over the rice, then top each serving with a tablespoon of yogurt.

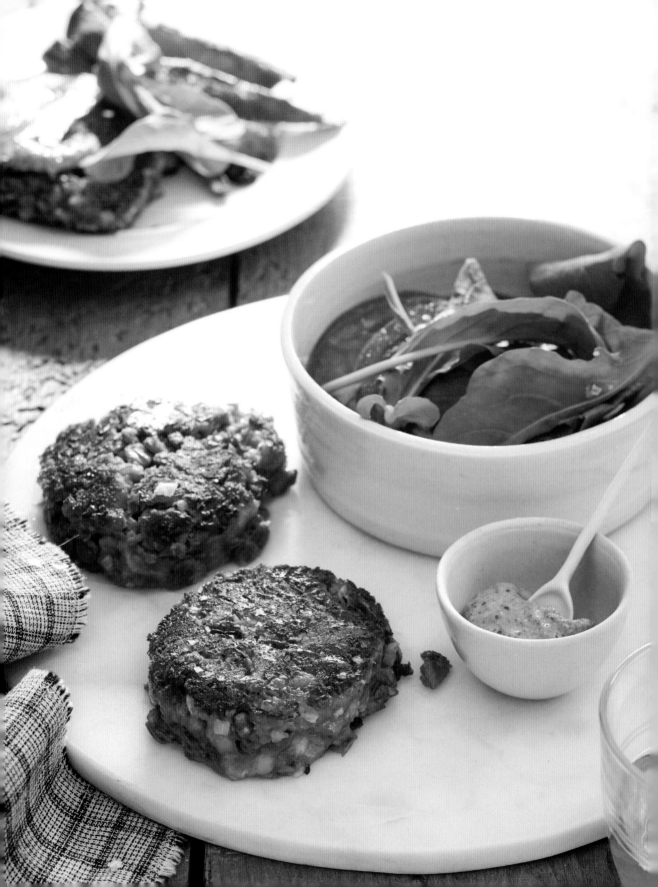

LENTIL VEGGIE BURGERS

Makes 8 patties

I love these burgers, based on a recipe from Health.com! The smokiness of the Cheddar still scratches that burger itch, even when you're not eating meat. And the lentils give you a lot of protein and good carb energy. I prefer to eat these burgers without the bun because the patties are so filling on their own. One note: They're a little tricky to flip in the pan because they can fall apart easily—so flip 'em quickly! And don't worry: even if they're not pretty, they taste delish. Make these along with Baked Sweet Potato Fries (page 95) if you want my version of a Big Mac with fries!

- 1 cup dried lentils, rinsed
- 2 bay leaves
- 2½ cups water
- 1 teaspoon olive oil
- 1 cup finely chopped onion
- ½ cup finely chopped carrot
- 1 cup shredded smoked Cheddar cheese (4 ounces)
- ½ cup breadcrumbs
- 2 teaspoons chopped fresh thyme
- 1¼ teaspoons salt
- ¾ teaspoon garlic powder
- ¾ teaspoon paprika
- ½ teaspoon freshly ground black pepper
- ¼ teaspoon cayenne pepper
- 3 large egg whites, lightly beaten
- Nonstick cooking spray
- 2 tablespoons plus 2 teaspoons stone-ground mustard
- 8 (2-ounce) whole wheat sandwich buns, toasted
- 1 large tomato, cut into ¼-inch-thick slices (about 8 slices)
- 2 cups arugula leaves

Place the lentils and bay leaves in a medium saucepan with 2½ cups of water and bring to a boil. Cover, reduce the heat, and simmer for 40 minutes, or until the lentils are tender. Drain, making sure you discard the bay leaves. Transfer the lentils to a large bowl and partially mash them with a fork or potato masher. Let them cool slightly.

continues

continued

Heat the oil in a medium nonstick skillet over medium-high heat. Add the on-ion and carrot and sauté for 5 minutes, or until tender. Let them cool slightly, then stir them into the lentils.

Add the cheese, breadcrumbs, thyme, salt, garlic powder, paprika, black pep-per, cayenne, and egg whites to the lentils and stir well to combine. Cover the mix with plastic wrap or foil and chill for 45 minutes in the fridge.

Divide the mixture into eight equal portions, shaping each into a ½-inch-thick patty.

Coat a grill pan with cooking spray and heat it over medium-high heat. Add half of the patties and cook for 5 minutes on each side, or until browned (remember to flip quickly and with confidence!). Repeat with the remaining patties.

To serve, spread a teaspoon of mustard on the top half of each bun. Place a patty on the bottom half and top with 1 tomato slice, ¼ cup arugula, and natch, the top half of the bun. Dinner's on!

SPAGHETTI WITH
TURKEY MEATBALLS & SAUCE

Makes 4 to 6 servings

Spaghetti is my favorite food. Like, beyond favorite. Desert island favorite. Last meal before the electric chair favorite. Kat and I had to go to Italy for some promotional work for our show, but really, we just wanted to eat spaghetti in Milan.

One of the reasons I fell for Michael was because, on our first Thanksgiving together, instead of turkey he made the special Sunday sauce that his grandma had learned from Italian immigrants in the South Philly neighborhood where she raised his dad.

Can you tell I have very warm feelings about spaghetti? For this recipe I included a version of his sauce that's just as delicious but much faster and easier to make.

These turkey meatballs, based on a recipe from Tia Mowry, are a winner because you can make a batch and keep them in your fridge or freezer, heating them as you need them. They are great for adding protein to your lunch or as a quick snack when you need to fill your stomach. And, of course, they're made for heaping on top of spaghetti.

By the way, if you're staying away from pasta, you can make this dish with steamed spaghetti squash instead, which has a noodle-ish consistency and is completely delish.

FOR THE MEATBALLS:

(Makes about 20 small meatballs)
- ½ cup old-fashioned oats
- ½ cup dairy milk of your choice
- ½ yellow onion, finely chopped
- ½ cup fresh baby spinach leaves, chopped
- ¼ cup grated Parmesan cheese
- 1 teaspoon kosher salt
- ½ teaspoon freshly ground black pepper
- 2 garlic cloves, grated
- 1 large egg
- 1 pound ground turkey
- 4 to 8 tablespoons olive oil

FOR THE SPAGHETTI AND SAUCE:

- 1 (28-ounce) can crushed tomatoes
- 2 tablespoons tomato paste
- 1 tablespoon chopped fresh oregano
- 1 teaspoon kosher salt, plus as needed for the pasta water
- ½ teaspoon freshly ground black pepper
- 2 garlic cloves, chopped
- 3 tablespoons red wine (optional)
- 1 teaspoon red pepper flakes (if you want to spice it up; optional)
- 1 pound spaghetti, cooked, or contents of 1 medium spaghetti squash, steamed

Chopped fresh parsley, for garnish
Chopped fresh basil, for garnish
Grated Parmesan cheese, for garnish

continues

continued

For the meatballs:

Add the oats to a blender and pulse a few times. It should look a little like breadcrumbs. Add the oats and milk to a small bowl and set aside.

Add the onions, spinach, Parmesan, salt, pepper, garlic, and egg to a large bowl and mix it all up. Add your oat mixture and combine. Finally, add the turkey and gently fold it into the wet mixture (make sure not to overmix!). Form the mixture into bite-size balls (you can use a small cookie scoop if you insist on matching-size meatballs).

Heat 4 tablespoons of the oil in a large pot. Add half of the meatballs and brown them on all sides (this will take about 5 to 7 minutes). Now repeat with the second batch, adding more oil if you need it. Set the meatballs aside but hold on to the pot for the sauce.

For the spaghetti and sauce:

Add the tomatoes, tomato paste, oregano, salt, pepper, and garlic to the pot and stir. Bring the sauce to a boil, then reduce the heat, cover, and let the sauce simmer for about 10 minutes. Gently add the browned meatballs to the sauce. Simmer, covered, until the meatballs are cooked through, another 10 to 15 minutes. If you want to give the sauce some richer flavor and a little bit of extra heat, add the red wine and pepper flakes right at the end, during the last 2 minutes of cooking.

Meanwhile, bring a large pot of water to a boil. Season the water with a generous pinch of salt. Add the spaghetti and cook until al dente, about 8 minutes. Drain and put the noodles back in the pot. Stir them with a ladle or two of sauce to keep them from sticking.

Plate the spaghetti and meatballs and ladle the remaining sauce over everything. Garnish with parsley, basil, and Parmesan. Serve hot and try not to inhale all at once.

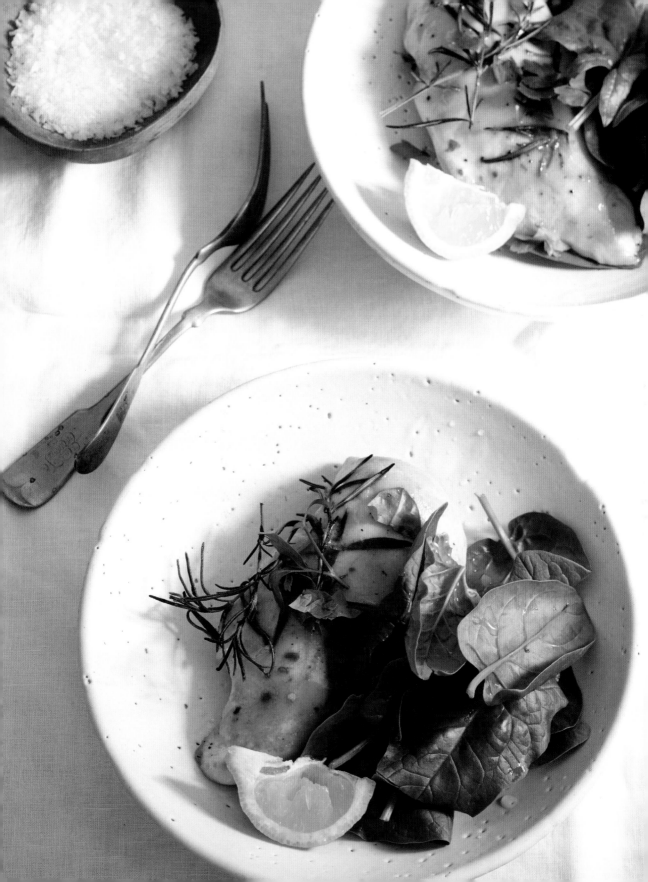

NO-FRILLS "GOURMET" CHICKEN

Makes 2 to 4 servings

This is a classic, simple recipe that is super healthy. Make this one when you have a date coming over for dinner or you want to impress any guest—it makes people who aren't expert cooks seem like they are. I like it because I don't have to think about dinner when I get home from work late—I just throw four breasts in the oven and I'm good to go, with leftovers for tomorrow.

    2 teaspoons kosher salt
    2 to 4 boneless, skinless chicken breasts
    ⅓ cup olive oil
    ⅓ cup freshly squeezed lemon juice (about 2 lemons)
    3 tablespoons honey
    2 tablespoons Dijon mustard
    ⅛ teaspoon freshly ground black pepper
    ¼ teaspoon red pepper flakes
    4 to 5 rosemary sprigs
    Chopped fresh parsley, for garnish
    Fresh spinach or arugula, for serving

Preheat the oven to 450°F.

Sprinkle salt on top of the chicken breasts and arrange them on a baking sheet.

In a small bowl, whisk together the olive oil, lemon juice, honey, mustard, black pepper, and pepper flakes. Pour the mixture on top of the chicken, using your hands to make sure it's slathered all over. Press rosemary sprigs all over the place.

Bake for 35 minutes, or until the chicken is no longer pink inside.

Garnish with parsley and serve on a bed of spinach or arugula.

BAKED (NOT FRIED!) FALAFEL
WITH SPICY YOGURT DIP

Makes 2 to 4 servings

Every once in a while I have a crazy craving for fried food . . . and I've finally figured out a way around it. The secret? Almost anything you need to fry (chicken, french fries, zucchini) can be baked in the oven instead—and still have that nice, crispy coating that you crave.

I adapted this recipe from the website How Sweet It Is (howsweeteats.com). Jessica Merchant, who runs the site, also wrote a cookbook called *Seriously Delish*, and I like that she doesn't take herself too seriously. She's passionate about food but open to experimentation and willing to make mistakes on the way to a great meal. Her baked falafel is a tasty vegetarian option that you can use as a main dish or a delicious snack, and you won't miss the way your hair smells after you fry something one bit. And remember, you can also use my Yummy Hummus recipe (page 67) as an alternative dip.

FOR THE FALAFEL:

- 2 (15-ounce) cans chickpeas, drained and rinsed
- 4 garlic cloves, chopped
- 4 scallions, sliced (green part only)
- 1 large egg
- Juice of 1 lemon
- ⅓ cup chopped fresh parsley
- ⅓ cup chopped fresh cilantro
- 1 tablespoon olive oil
- 1 teaspoon salt
- 1 teaspoon freshly ground black pepper
- ½ teaspoon ground cumin
- ½ teaspoon smoked paprika
- ¼ cup whole wheat or all-purpose flour
- 1 teaspoon baking powder

FOR THE DIP:

- ½ cup low-fat or nonfat plain Greek yogurt
- 1 cup crumbled feta cheese
- 1½ tablespoons olive oil
- ¼ teaspoon salt
- ¼ teaspoon freshly ground black pepper
- ⅛ teaspoon cayenne pepper
- Chopped fresh parsley, for garnish
- Red pepper flakes, for garnish

continues

continued

Preheat the oven to 400°F.

In a blender (preferably a Vitamix or other high-powered blender), combine the chickpeas, garlic, scallions, egg, lemon juice, parsley, cilantro, oil, salt, pepper, cumin, and paprika. Pulse until the mixture is combined but still crumbly, not smooth. Add half of the flour and baking powder and pulse a few more times until fully combined. Repeat with the remaining flour and baking powder.

Scoop out about 2 tablespoons' worth of the falafel mixture and form it into a small patty or ball. Look, falafel! Repeat, repeat. Place the balls on an oiled or parchment-lined baking sheet and bake them for 20 minutes. They should be a little crispy on top and cooked all the way through.

While the falafel is baking, clean your blender and add all the ingredients for the dip. Pulse until blended. Garnish with parsley and a sprinkle of red pepper flakes. Serve with the falafel.

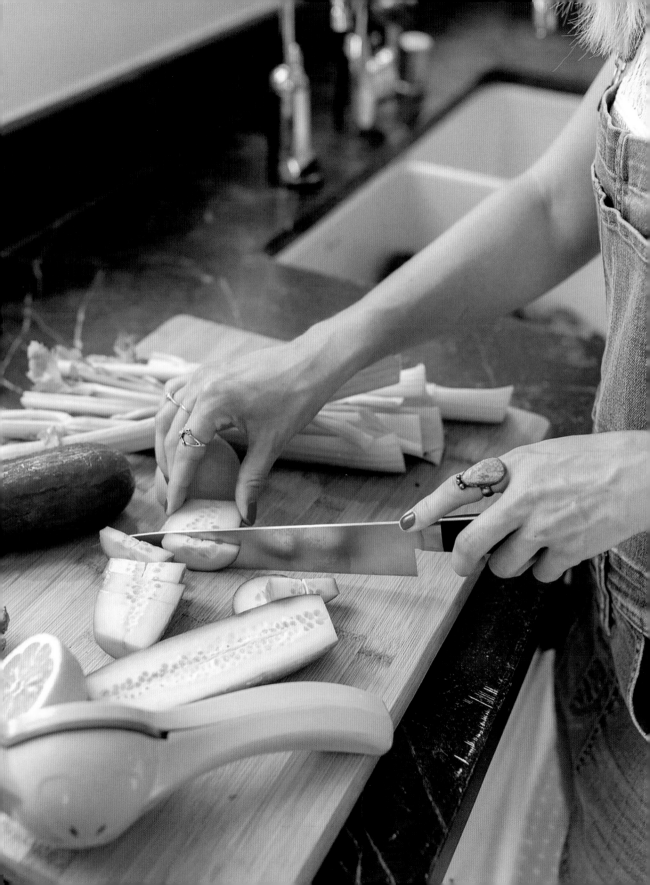

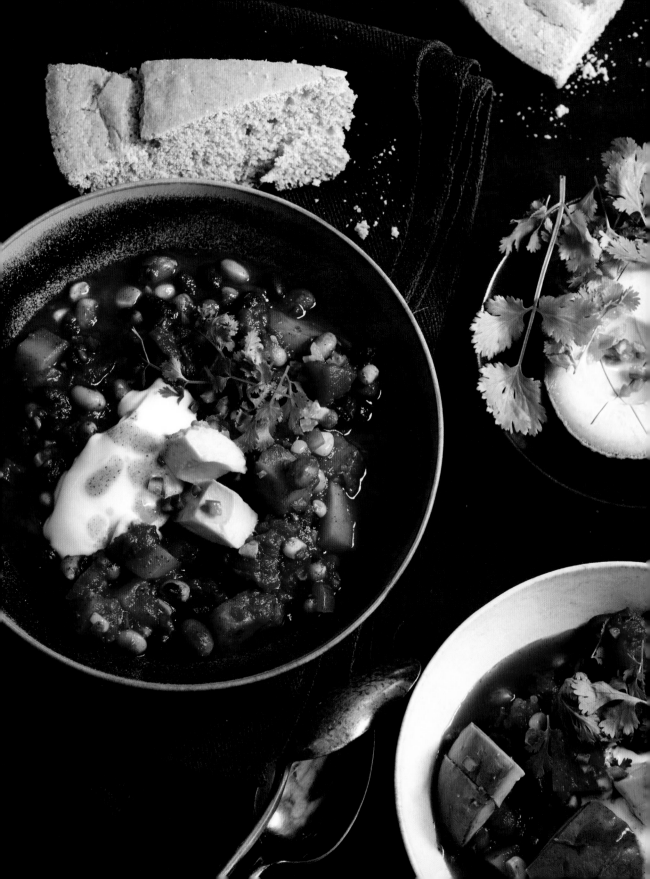

CHAPTER 6

INVITE OTHERS:
CROWD-PLEASING MEALS

You've made small changes. You've started cooking and have figured out how to maximize meals. Now let's explore the next natural step: the joy of food and friendship—inviting others to be a part of your eating experience!

STRESSED ABOUT EATING OUT?

Eating socially has its ups and its downs. Ups: the delight of getting friends together to enjoy something you've made. Downs: the strategic and emotional challenges of restaurants and big family gatherings, from finding something you want to eat on the menu to dismissing others' commentary about what you order.

If you're going to eat out, do a little reconnaissance first to make sure you'll be able to eat something that works for you. If you're going to a restaurant, check its website or call ahead to ask what's on the menu. If you're invited over to someone's house, you can ask what's going to be served (tell the host it's not a big deal, but you have some dietary restrictions) or offer to bring something you know you'll want to eat. If you want a little more control, or if you love throwing a party (like I do), then invite everyone over to your place. Involving others in your appreciation for the new foods you're eating is the next step in your process. That means making sure there's going to be food that *you* like to eat and things *you* like to prepare. Give yourself some added time for shopping, prepping, and setting up. Try to enjoy yourself while it's all happening—and then ask your friends to help with the cleanup!

GROUPS

The recipes that follow fall into three categories: Groups, Soups, and Desserts. They're organized this way because they sound good together, and also because they're all naturally well suited for feeding a crowd. Group recipes yield a large number of servings, so you can either dole them out or freeze leftovers to keep yourself stocked for future meals. Soups are perfect for serving when you have people over for an actual meal (as opposed to finger foods), and serving soup makes you look like a polished pro—which at this point, you are! And just like the group recipes, you can cook a lot up front and save some servings in the freezer for later. Desserts, well, that should need no explanation—what better reason to make a sweet, delicious treat than to share it!

MICHAEL'S "RING OF FIRE" CHILI
(THE VEGAN VERSION)

Makes 20 to 25 servings

Here's the thing about chili: Everyone does it her own way. That's why there are so many chili cook-offs! Michael and I like cooking "by feel," meaning we can eyeball what goes into a dish and adjust the seasoning as we go. It's way more fun that way! But I realize that for some of you kitchen novices, it might be helpful to have actual measurements. Use this recipe as a guide, and as you get more comfortable trusting your instincts, start to improvise—add different spices in different amounts or heap in all kinds of other veggies. The best part of this dish is that every batch tastes different.

The squash was Michael's greatest inspiration for veggie chili. It's his go-to meat substitute, and for good reason in chili: The sweetness of the squash really plays off the heat of the spices. He's no fan of red kidney beans—they're way too school cafeteria for Michael's taste—so he recommends using pinto, white, black, or pink beans or black-eyed peas instead. He likes Herb-Ox bouillon cubes and Gebhardt's Eagle Brand chili powder, but any good-quality chili powder will do. If you have a local spice shop nearby (we swear by the Spice Station in LA), pick up your chili powder there! And your cumin, too—it's the spice that makes chili, chili. Initially, you'll only need to put in a portion of the spices, then you can continue to add more spices and "heat" to your taste as your chili cooks.

This recipe feeds twenty to twenty-five people, so feel free to halve it if you don't want to make such a big batch (though it freezes really nicely). Also, it always tastes better the next day, so it's a great dish to make ahead.

I've included a recipe for gluten-free cornbread, which is the perfect accompaniment once you've entered THE RING OF FIRE (explosion noise here!).

continues

Canned beans are easiest, but if you wanna get LEGIT, here's an excellent bean recipe. (Once cooked, the beans can be added directly to the chili.):

Soak the beans of your choice (pinto, white, black, pink, etc.) in water for the amount of time specified on the package, or overnight. (Every bag of dried beans has preparation/cooking instructions printed on it. One type of bean may differ from another, so follow the instructions printed on the bag of beans you have.) Drain. Add the soaked beans, a whole peeled onion, a large peeled garlic clove, and 2 tablespoons dried oregano to a large pot filled with enough water to cover everything. Cook as directed until the beans are tender but not mushy. Remove the onion and garlic before serving.

continued

Olive oil, for generously coating skillet

4 cups finely chopped onion

10 to 12 large garlic cloves, finely chopped

6 cups canned whole peeled tomatoes

3 cups tomato purée

2 cups crushed tomatoes

7 cups cubed butternut squash, 1½- to 2-inch cubes

4 large portobello mushroom caps, cut into ½- to 1-inch cubes

2 cobs' worth of sweet corn

2 (15.5-ounce) cans black beans (see note), drained and rinsed

2 (15.5-ounce) cans black-eyed peas (see note), drained and rinsed

2 (15.5-ounce) cans pinto beans (see note), drained and rinsed

¼ cup salt, or 6 vegan bouillon cubes

2 cups good-quality chili powder

5 teaspoons dried oregano

2 tablespoons freshly ground black pepper

1 teaspoon dried rosemary

4 to 6 teaspoons ground cumin

2 to 3 cups dry red wine (optional)

2 to 3 teaspoons Pickapeppa Sauce or vegan Worcestershire sauce

1 bell pepper (any color), cored, seeded, and finely chopped

4 to 8 medium-size jalapeño peppers, seeded (or not, fire eaters) and finely chopped

1 to 6 serrano chiles, finely chopped (optional; if you can't take the heat, use only the jalapeños)

½ to 1 habanero chile, finely chopped (WARNING: OPTIONAL! THIS CHILE PEPPER IS ONE OF THE HOTTEST, AND IT IS ONLY TO BE USED BY THOSE WHO LIKE IT *VERY* HOT!)

2 tablespoons cayenne pepper

Chipotle chili powder, red pepper flakes, or any other crushed peppers, to taste

Your favorite hot sauce (Tabasco, Tapatío, Cholula, Frank's, etc.), to taste

2 recipes Gluten-Free Cornbread (recipe follows)

Heat the olive oil in a large skillet over medium-high heat and add the onions. Sauté until golden but not too brown (or burnt!). Add the garlic in the last few minutes.

Chop the peeled tomatoes and add them to the pan, including their liquid. Add the tomato purée and crushed tomatoes and cook for a minute or two. Stir in the remaining ingredients, adding the spices, chile peppers, and hot sauce to taste.

Simmer for as little as 1 hour but no more than 2. Serve with cornbread.

OPTIONAL: For additional flavor, finely chop the cooked onion and garlic, then mix them back into the beans before serving.

GLUTEN-FREE CORNBREAD

Makes 12 pieces

To go with your chili—or anytime. There are lots of gluten-free cornbread recipes out there, but I like this one because it's not all that complicated, and the final product is sooo tasty. This has a little bit of a sweet vibe, but I like to tang it up a smidge by adding a few teaspoons of chopped jalapeño to the mix (you know me, I like everything spicy). You can make it in a skillet to go old-school, but a baking dish will work just as well.

     6 tablespoons unsalted butter, divided
  1½ cups gluten-free all-purpose flour
  1½ cups gluten-free cornmeal
   ⅓ cup granulated sugar
     2 teaspoons baking powder
     1 teaspoon baking soda
     1 teaspoon salt
     2 large eggs, or ½ cup egg substitute
  1½ cups dairy or nondairy milk of your choice (I like unsweetened almond or
        coconut milk in this recipe)
        Few teaspoons chopped jalapeño pepper (optional)
     2 tablespoons honey, for serving

Preheat the oven to 400°F. Grease a medium-size cast-iron skillet or an 8 x 8-inch baking dish with just enough butter to coat the pan. Let the pan warm up inside the oven while you make the cornbread. Melt the remaining butter and set aside to cool slightly.

Mix the flour, cornmeal, sugar, baking powder, baking soda, and salt in a large bowl until well combined.

In a separate bowl, whisk together the eggs and milk, then add the cooled melted butter to the mixture.

Combine all the ingredients, including the jalapeños, if using, and mix well with a wooden spoon or spatula. It doesn't need to be smooth and silky. Pour the batter into the heated skillet or baking dish.

Lower the oven temperature to 350°F and bake the cornbread for 30 to 40 minutes, or until a toothpick inserted in the center comes out clean. Drizzle with honey before serving.

ALMOST-AUTHENTIC VEGETARIAN ENCHILADA CASSEROLE

Makes 5 to 6 servings

This dish is based on a vegetarian recipe that I love from Oh She Glows (ohsheglows .com), and we make it for dinner a whole bunch. It's not the healthiest dish, but we modify it by using rice pasta instead of white pasta. You can also make it with brown rice instead of pasta and make it more like a burrito filling or a burrito bowl. If you're trying to keep it real, you can go light on the cheese (or use nondairy cheese) and stay away from the Mexican toppings like sour cream . . . but mmm-hmm they taste so good. This is really the perfect thing to make when you're craving Taco Bell!

3½ cups fusilli or rice pasta (about 8 ounces), or 1 cup cooked brown rice

1 teaspoon olive oil

1 red onion, chopped

1 medium-size jalapeño pepper, seeded and chopped (see note on page 48)

3 bell peppers (any color combo), cored, seeded, and chopped

1 to 3 tablespoons taco seasoning mix

1 (15-ounce) can black beans, drained and rinsed, or 2 cups cooked (see note on page 129)

1½ to 2 cups Super Enchilada Sauce (recipe follows) or store-bought, divided

⅓ to ½ cup Mexican cheese blend or Cheddar, plus more for sprinkling on top

1 cup chopped scallions (green part only)

Salt and freshly ground black pepper, to taste

2 dozen tortilla chips (about 2 handfuls), crushed, plus whole chips for serving

Chopped avocado, salsa, sour cream (any of your favorite Mexican-style toppings), for garnish

Preheat the oven to 350°F and have a 2-quart casserole dish handy.

Bring a large pot of water to a boil and add the pasta. Cook for 7 to 8 minutes; it should still be a little undercooked, as you don't want it to get mushy when you bake it in the casserole. Drain the pasta and rinse with cold water to stop the cooking process.

In a large skillet, heat the oil over medium heat and add the onion, jalapeño, and peppers. Cook for about 7 to 8 minutes, or until the veggies are soft.

continues

continued

Sprinkle in the taco seasoning to taste and add the black beans and 1 cup of the enchilada sauce. Stir and cook for another 5 minutes.

Stir in the cheese, pasta or cooked brown rice, and scallions. Taste and adjust the seasoning with salt and pepper, if necessary.

Spread ½ cup of the enchilada sauce over the bottom of the casserole dish. Scoop the pasta mixture into the dish and spread out evenly. Pour ½ cup of the enchilada sauce on top, if desired. Sprinkle with cheese.

Bake for 15 to 20 minutes, or until heated through. Garnish with the crushed chips, avocado, salsa, and sour cream (if you're going for it) just before serving. Add some whole chips on the side for scooping.

SUPER ENCHILADA SAUCE

Makes 2 cups

This sauce packs a lot of tomato flavor and really gives extra dimension to the enchiladas. I like my sauce kind of thick, but you can always add water to thin it out. No surprise that I also like it a little spicy, but you can go lighter on the heat if you want to. (But c'mon! Heat is good for your digestion!) You can prepare the sauce a day or so before you make your enchiladas and keep it refrigerated. That way you have one less thing to worry about while you're cooking your main dish.

    2 tablespoons extra-virgin olive oil
    1 tablespoon all-purpose flour
    2 tablespoons chili powder
    1 teaspoon ground cumin
    ¼ teaspoon cayenne pepper
    ¾ teaspoon garlic powder
    ½ teaspoon onion powder
    2 (8-ounce) cans tomato paste
    1 cup plus ¼ cup water (more if you'd like a sauce that's not as thick)
    Salt and freshly ground black pepper, to taste

In a small bowl, whisk together the oil, flour, and chili powder until it's clump-free. Transfer the mixture to a small pot and cook over medium heat for a couple of minutes, whisking constantly.

In the same bowl, mix the cumin, cayenne, garlic powder, and onion powder. Whisk this into the mixture in the pot until completely smooth and then whisk in the tomato paste and water (start with 1 cup and add ¼ cup if a thinner sauce is desired). Continue whisking until saucy-looking.

Simmer the sauce over medium-low heat for 10 to 15 minutes, whisking about every 5 minutes. Add salt and pepper to taste and adjust seasonings if necessary.

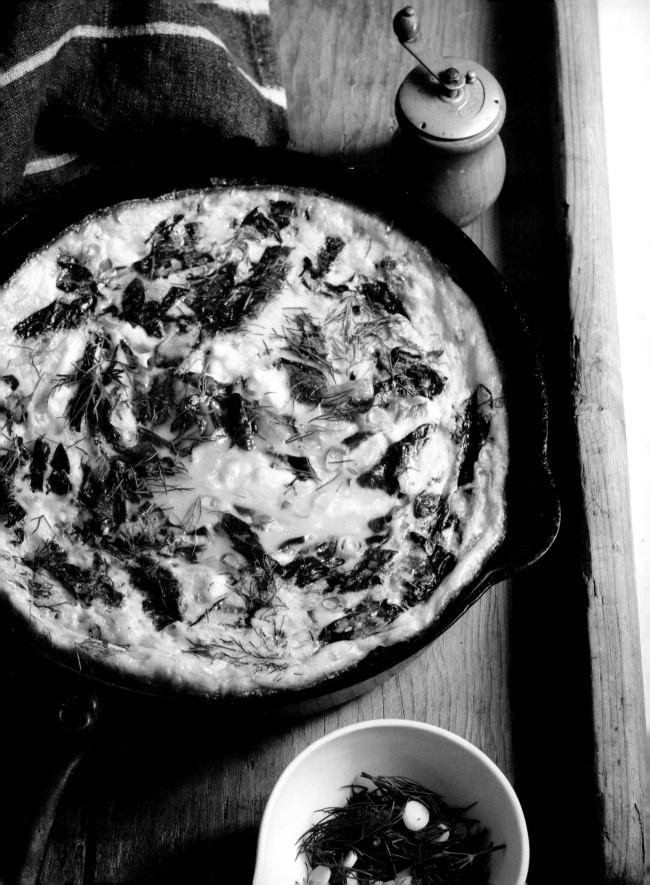

ANYTHING GOES FRITTATA

Makes 4 to 6 servings

When I'm looking to feed a big group of people, I think frittata. This quiche-omelet mashup can be served hot or cold, and you can toss in almost any ingredients—so it puts those last few veggies left in the bin to good use. It's a great brunch option but works equally well for lunch and dinner. All that's really involved is precooking your veggie mix-ins (and in the case of watery guys like tomatoes or mushrooms, ditching as much of that moisture as possible so your frittata doesn't get soggy), stirring them into beaten eggs, and then baking. In addition to veggies, consider including smoked salmon or sausage (if you're a meat eater)—just not both at the same time. Smoked salmon and sausage frittata? That's a NO.

You can make and serve this in a cast-iron skillet for that rustic look. Or you can use an ovenproof skillet or a 2-quart baking dish. Make two at a time for a larger group.

FRITTATA BASE:

- 3 tablespoons olive oil
- ½ cup diced onion
- 8 large eggs
- ½ cup whole milk (you need this for fluffiness, so that's why whole milk is your best bet)
- ¾ teaspoon salt
- ¼ teaspoon freshly ground black pepper

MAKE IT GREEK:

- 6 cups baby spinach, dried well
- ½ cup crumbled feta cheese
- 2 tablespoons chopped fresh dill
- 2 tablespoons sliced scallions (green part only)
- ½ cup chopped red bell pepper (optional)
- 2 ounces shredded mozzarella cheese (optional)

Preheat the oven to 350°F.

In a 10-inch ovenproof skillet or 2-quart baking dish, heat the oil over medium-high heat. Add the onion and cook until soft, about 5 minutes.

In a bowl, beat the eggs just enough to mix the whites and yolks, but don't overblend. Add the milk, salt, and pepper and whisk until just combined.

Time to go Greek: Add the spinach, feta, dill, and scallions to the egg mixture, along with the bell pepper, if using. (And I recommend you do—it's great for taste and color!)

Pour the mixture over the onions in that warm baking dish/skillet on the stove. Stir to combine and cook, undisturbed, for 5 to 7 minutes, or until the edges begin to pull away from the pan. Then put the whole thing in the oven for 16 to 18 minutes.

Do not overcook your frittata! I know you'll want it to look browned on top, but that means it's overcooked. Go crazy and sprinkle a little mozzarella on top instead before you serve.

SOUPS

As I mentioned, these recipes yield a lot of soup. If you aren't serving the soup to friends, you can refrigerate leftovers or freeze them in glass bowls with fitted lids, so all you need to do is heat and eat. I like Pyrex, but I've also used lower-end brands to save $. Costco has great deals on glassware, so I don't worry about bringing my soup to work for lunch, knowing I may forget the bowl there.

BIG GROUP LENTIL SOUP

Makes 4 to 6 servings

Michael has a friend, Stelani, who is Greek, and this is her mother's lentil soup recipe. (Michael—you did get permission to share this one, right?) It's hard to put the taste into words, but it's homey and warm and fragrant. It's not made with cream, but it tastes like a creamy soup—that's the magic of the lentils.

- ⅓ cup olive oil
- 1 Vidalia onion, chopped
- 1 bulb fresh garlic, chopped
- 1 tablespoon garlic powder
- Salt, to taste
- 1 teaspoon dried oregano, or more to taste
- 1 teaspoon dried basil, or more to taste
- 1 teaspoon dried or fresh parsley, or more to taste
- 1 chicken bouillon cube or packet
- 1 small strip of orange peel, fresh or dried
- 1 (28-ounce) can whole peeled San Marzano tomatoes
- 1 (16-ounce) bag dried lentils, rinsed
- 7 to 8 bay leaves

In a large stew pot over medium heat, combine the oil, onion, garlic, garlic powder, salt, oregano, basil, parsley, bouillon, and orange peel. Cook until the onions are almost translucent, 5 to 6 minutes. Add the tomatoes and their juices, using your spoon to break them into smaller pieces and release their liquid.

Stir in the lentils and add just enough water to cover the ingredients. Bring to a boil over high heat, then reduce to a simmer. Add the bay leaves. Continue simmering until the lentils are fully cooked, about 5 to 7 minutes, adding more water if necessary. Taste as the lentils cook and adjust the seasoning if desired.

Remove the bay leaves and orange peel, then transfer the pot to the fridge and let sit covered overnight (the flavors get better as the stew sits). Don't be tempted to take the bay leaves or orange peel out later—they'll make the stew bitter.

TWO TOMATO SOUPS

I am such a soup person, but I wasn't always. I did, however, have a childhood obsession with tomato soup—at least asking about it. Family lore has it that every day when I was little, I would ask my babysitter, "Do you have tomato soup?" Then she would say, "Yes. Do you want some?" And I'd say, "Nope." I don't know why—it was just one of those ongoing family jokes. But I really missed out! My curiosity finally got the best of me at the ripe old age of twenty-five, when I tried tomato soup for the first time in a Nordstrom café. It changed my life. Tomato soup is just so comforting. That warm, creamy taste makes you think of rainy days and grilled cheese . . . it gives you the feeling of home.

Here are two recipes for tomato soup, one vegan and one not. The NOT vegan version comes from Martha Stewart, who appeared on our show in its first season. I am legendarily potty-mouthed on our set, but when Martha showed up, everyone teased me for being so prim and proper. The vegan version is a slight modification of a recipe I found on Blissful Basil (blissfulbasil.com), a fantastic website where vegan blogger Ashley Melillo offers wonderful ideas for plant-based eating. The cauliflower base and nutritional yeast make the soup hearty enough for a meal.

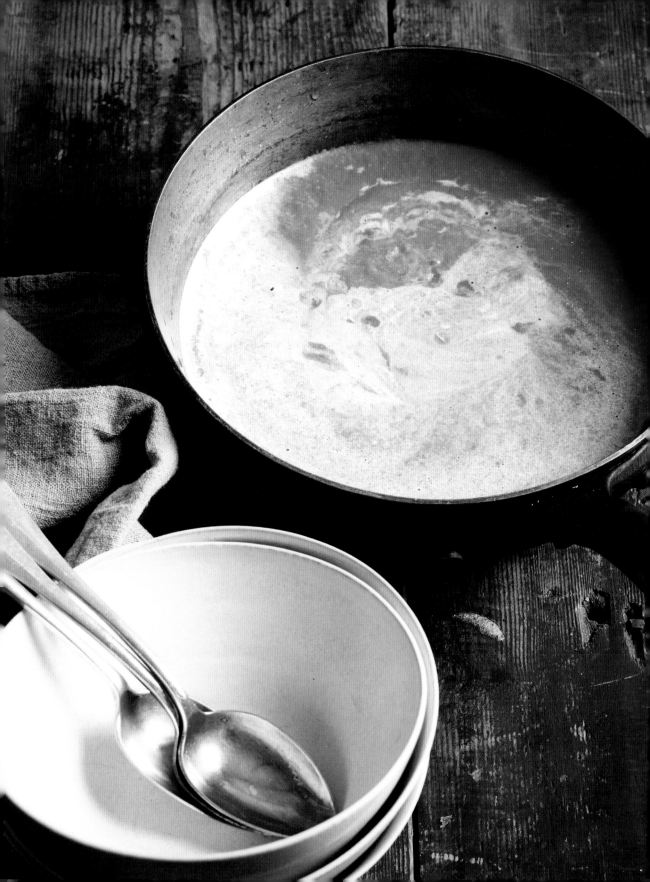

MARTHA STEWART'S (NON-VEGAN) TOMATO SOUP

Makes 6 servings

  2 tablespoons unsalted butter
  1 onion, coarsely chopped
  1 to 2 garlic cloves (optional)
  2 (14-ounce) cans whole peeled tomatoes
1½ cups chicken stock or water
    Coarse salt and freshly ground black pepper, to taste
  ½ cup heavy cream (optional)

Melt the butter in a medium stockpot over medium heat. Cook the onion and garlic, if using, stirring constantly, until they're soft and translucent, about 3 minutes.

Add the tomatoes and their juices, plus the stock. Season with salt and pepper and bring to a boil, then lower the heat and simmer for 10 minutes.

Working in batches, transfer the tomato mixture to a blender. Purée the tomato mixture, making sure your blender is completely covered or it will splatter everywhere. You can use a kitchen towel to cover the lid, if necessary. (Alternatively, blend the soup in the pot using an immersion blender.)

Return the puréed soup to a pot and set over low heat. Whisk in the cream, if using, and season with salt and pepper. Serve the soup immediately or let it cool before transferring it to a covered container to refrigerate or freeze. Reheat it over medium heat.

HEARTY VEGAN TOMATO SOUP

Makes 6 servings

3 tablespoons extra-virgin olive oil, plus more for serving
4 garlic cloves, minced
1 medium yellow onion, diced
1 red bell pepper, cored, seeded, and roughly chopped
2 (28-ounce) cans whole peeled tomatoes
1 small head cauliflower, roughly chopped
1 teaspoon dried oregano
1 teaspoon dried basil
Pinch of red pepper flakes (optional)
3 tablespoons nutritional yeast flakes
Sea salt, to taste
Chopped fresh basil, for garnish (optional)

Heat the oil in a large pot over medium heat. Add the garlic and onion and cook for about 5 minutes, or until they're nice and tender. Add the bell pepper and cook for another 2 minutes—make sure no seeds get in there or you'll have waaay too much heat! Stir in the tomatoes and their juices, cauliflower, oregano, dried basil, and pepper flakes, if using (of course, *I'm* using them). Make sure the cauliflower is coated in the tomato sauce; it will cook down a bit eventually.

Bring the mixture to a boil. Reduce the heat, cover, and allow it to simmer for about 25 minutes. Turn off the heat.

Working in batches if necessary, pour the mixture into your blender (be careful; it's still hot!) and blend until completely smooth. Return the soup to the pot. (Alternatively, blend the soup in the pot using an immersion blender.)

Add the nutritional yeast and season with salt to taste (try to go easy on the salt). Simmer on low for an additional 10 to 15 minutes, stirring occasionally. I like my tomato soup thick, but if it's too thick for your taste, add some water (no more than a cup) and stir until you reach the desired consistency.

Ladle the soup into bowls. For presentation and taste, I suggest that you drizzle each bowl with olive oil and sprinkle it with fresh basil.

FOOD FUN WITH FRIENDS

So what happens when you've slowly but surely changed your diet, but you still want to have a good food-and-cocktail-related time? Snacking your way through happy hour or staying out all night at the bar might not hold the same allure for you as it used to. Even meeting for coffee—especially if "coffee" was really just code for a sugary, caramel-y, creamy whipped drink-accino at the corner coffee shop—might not be appealing once you've discovered the joy of a Chococado Smoothie (page 49). Initially I found I was getting a little case of the lonelies as I began to embrace healthier, more sensible food choices. You might be in luck and have a lot of friends on board. (Research shows that it's easier to diet, exercise, and stick to other life-changing regimes if you do it with other like-minded people.) But when everyone else is still packing in the carbs and sugar, it can get lonely when you're living right. To keep yourself focused—but still in the social mix—here are some fun group activities that are good for you, and your friends, too.

Vegan Baking Party

Just like Xmas-cookie decorating, but healthier. There are great recipes at sites like Oh, Ladycakes (ohladycakes.com), C'est La Vegan (cestlavegan.com), and Elissa Goodman (elissagoodman.com)—and Oh She Glows (ohsheglows.com) has the best recipes of them all! My BFF Alisha, who was my roommate during college, has been vegan for years, and she swears by the site. Pumpkin gingerbread muffins, snickerdoodles, toffee cinnamon oatmeal cookie bars . . . baking fans will find lots to love here, along with delicious recipes for meals and sides.

Spice Shopping Spree

Take a friend shopping at a local spice shop—or better yet, buy some single spices at the shop, then have a get-together where everyone makes their own signature spice blends.

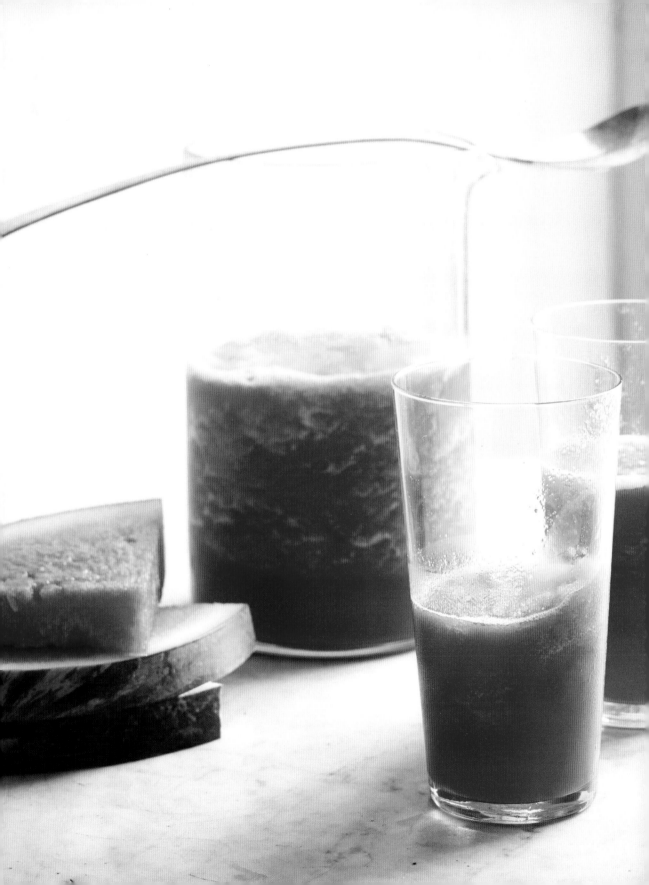

Chill Chili Party

Throw the ingredients for the chili recipe on page 129 in a pot and have a glass of organic wine with your gal pals while dinner cooks. Just remember to soak the beans the night before!

Skinny Cocktail Parties

The next time you have people over, put out pitchers of "skinny" (lower-sugar) or healthy (nonalcoholic) drinks instead of the usual beer, wine, and sugary mixers. Try some different fresh fruit juices and have a friend play bartender with these mixology creations.

O.J. (OH JOY) SPRITZER

Makes 2 servings

¼ cup orange juice (freshly squeezed is best)
¼ cup peach juice
1 cup seltzer or sparkling water
Lemon or lime slices, for garnish

Chill all ingredients before mixing. Pour into glasses (over ice, if you prefer), add citrus garnish, and say "Cheers!"

WATERMELON FREEZE

Makes 4 servings

3 cups chopped watermelon, chilled
1 cup coconut water
Squeeze of fresh lime juice
1 cup crushed ice

Put all the ingredients in a blender and blend until smooth.

DESSERTS

DESSERTS

Just because you're taking good care of your body doesn't mean you'll never enjoy another sweet treat. There are a lot of delicious *and* healthy options for dessert, including things you can bring to friends' homes, celebrations, or the breakroom at work so you're not suffering through yet another birthday party sponsored by Krispy Kreme.

I'm not the biggest dessert person—I'm more of a salty/savory junkie—but I'm reminded of my two-doughnut-a-day habit from UCLA every time I get a whiff of the doughnut place on my corner . . . it's dangerous! Sometimes you just can't ignore the voice in your head begging for something sweet. And when that happens, you have these recipes to scratch that itch. Just remember—they're still a treat, and not something I recommend indulging in every day. But when I do want something sugary and yummy, I go for one of these recipes.

Plus, baking is fun! When I bake, I get warm fuzzies thinking about being in the kitchen with my great aunt Meme, a liberal nun from upstate New York (the very same woman who would knit me potholders). In addition to being an expert crafter, she was the world's best cookie- and pie-maker. We'd bake on Christmas Day, then get up at 5 a.m. the day after to get stuff half off at Michael's. Makes me want to knit a potholder right this second. I promise you, even if the most complicated thing you've ever made is brownies out of a box, you'll be able to whip up your own delicious confections. Be patient and remember: Even the mistakes are delicious.

VEGAN TRUFFLES

Makes 12 to 16 truffles

A chocolate truffle is such a perfect little dessert, and the taste is totally decadent. You can personalize truffles in any way you want. Spice fans like me can add a ¼ teaspoon of cayenne and a teaspoon of cinnamon to the mix and end up with Tex-Mex truffles. Or you can keep your chocolate mix pure and roll your balls in chopped nuts to get super-crunch truffles. You can also get creative with herbs, spices, or dried fruit. This truffle 101 recipe will get you started.

- ¼ cup coconut milk
- 2 cups dark chocolate chips (70% cacao), vegan if preferred
- ¼ cup plus 2 tablespoons coconut oil
- ⅓ cup raw cacao powder, chopped nuts, or flaked coconut

Heat the coconut milk in a double boiler. (If you don't have a double boiler, you can simmer a few inches of water in a saucepan and then nestle a metal or glass bowl on top of it. Just make sure the bottom of the bowl isn't touching the water.) Stir in the chocolate chips and coconut oil until melted and well combined.

Transfer the mixture to a shallow bowl and refrigerate until completely cooled.

Use a spoon or melon baller to create your truffles, roll them in your palms to smooth, and roll each one in cacao powder, nuts, or coconut before transferring to a storage container. Your truffles will keep in the fridge for 2 to 3 weeks.

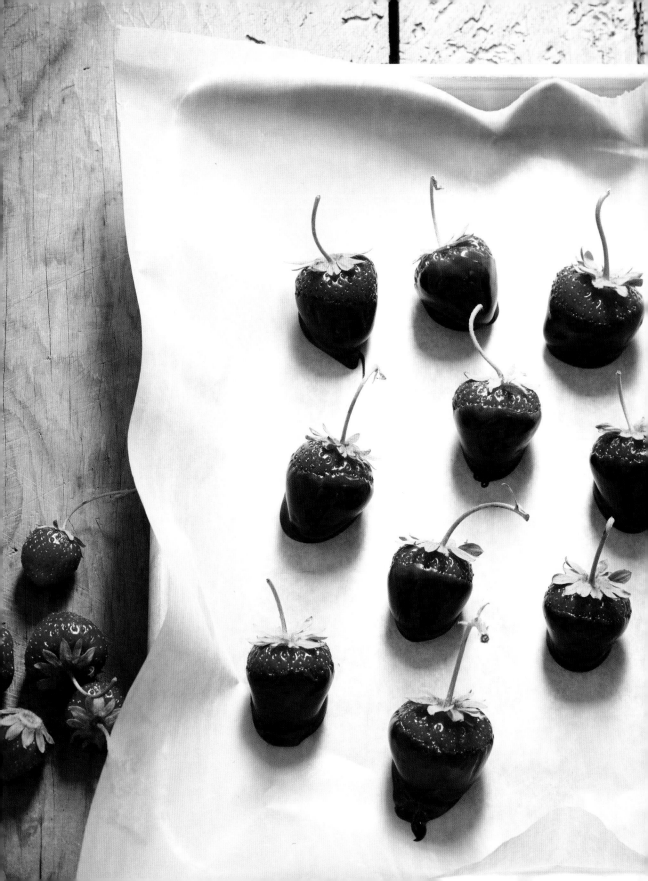

CHOCOLATE-COVERED FRUIT

Makes 12 servings

When vegan friends are over and hoping for something delicious to eat, I put out this dessert, which is my version of a fondue party. I love chocolate-covered fruit, especially because dark chocolate has a little bit of "good for you–ness" to it. (That's a scientific term.) Chocolate with a high percentage of cacao in it—70 percent or higher—makes you feel good by raising serotonin and endorphin levels in the brain, and it is filled with antioxidants and magnesium, which helps chill out your nerves and lower your heart rate. And don't even get me started on how great fruit is for you. (Hello, phytochemicals and antioxidants!) Feel free to sub in your favorites.

12 strawberries, with stems or skewered on toothpicks
½ cup dark chocolate chips (70% cacao), vegan if preferred

Line a baking sheet with waxed paper and wash and dry the strawberries.

Melt the chocolate in a double boiler. (If you don't have a double boiler, you can simmer a few inches of water in a saucepan and then nestle a metal or glass bowl on top of it. Just make sure the bottom of the bowl isn't touching the water.)

Holding the berries by their stem or toothpick, dip each one into the chocolate, then set it onto the baking sheet. Once all of your berries have been dipped, transfer the baking sheet to the refrigerator and let them cool completely (about 1 hour).

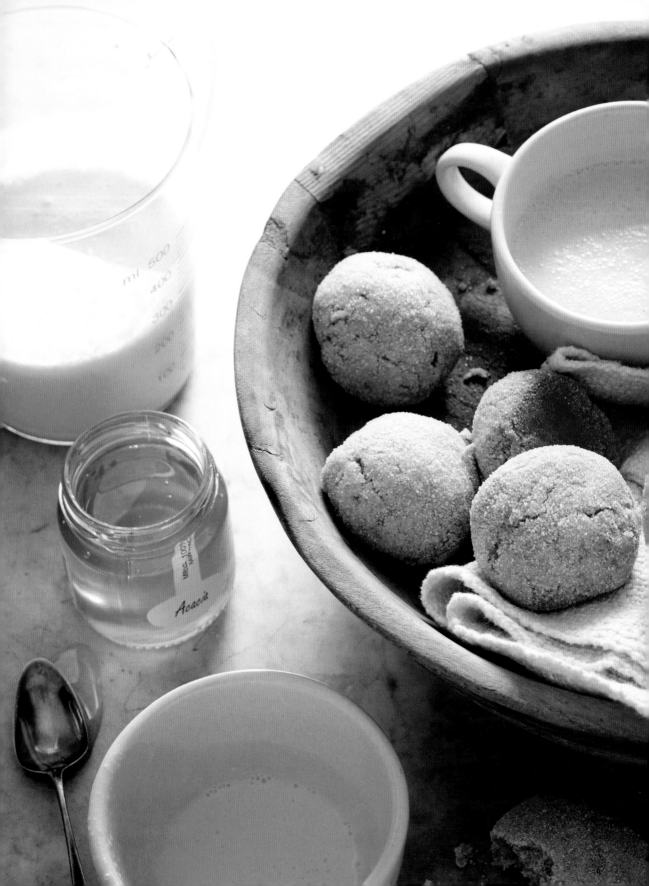

ANYTIME GINGER COOKIES

Makes 2 dozen cookies

These cookies are delicious year-round, but especially when the weather cools because ginger is a nice, warm spice. And they're just the things for holiday cookie swaps and gifts. This recipe makes about two dozen cookies, so feel free to freeze some of the dough for the next time you're in the mood for a fresh ginger cookie.

1½ cups all-purpose flour, plus as needed for shaping the dough
 1 cup whole wheat flour
 ¾ cup chopped crystallized ginger
 1 teaspoon baking powder
 ½ teaspoon baking soda
 ½ teaspoon salt
 ½ teaspoon ground ginger
1¼ cups granulated sugar, divided
 ½ cup unsweetened applesauce
 ¼ cup vegetable oil
 1 teaspoon grated lemon zest
 1 tablespoon freshly squeezed lemon juice
 ¼ teaspoon vanilla extract
   Nonstick cooking spray

In a large bowl, whisk together the flours, crystallized ginger, baking powder, baking soda, salt, and ground ginger.

In a medium bowl, combine 1 cup of the sugar with the applesauce, vegetable oil, lemon zest, lemon juice, and vanilla. Make a well in the center of the dry ingredients and pour the wet ingredients into the well. Stir just until combined, then cover the bowl with plastic wrap and chill the dough in the fridge for at least 1 hour.

Preheat the oven to 350°F. Coat two baking sheets with nonstick cooking spray.

Add the remaining ¼ cup sugar to a small shallow bowl. Lightly coat your hands with flour and shape the dough into 24 balls (about 2 tablespoons each; the dough will be sticky). Roll the balls in the sugar to coat and arrange them on the baking sheets at least 2 inches apart. Bake for 15 minutes, or until lightly browned. Cool for 1 minute on the pan, then transfer the cookies to wire racks to cool completely.

PEARS WITH ROSEMARY SUGAR

Makes 24 slices

You already know I'm a major rosemary fan, so I'm glad Real Simple came up with a way to enjoy it as a sweet accent, not a savory one. The great citrus flavor from the orange juice gives a little extra zing and brings out the flavor of the pear, which so often comes in second place to apples. Well, not anymore! Another bonus: You can whip up this dessert in minutes.

- 3 green Anjou pears
- ¼ cup freshly squeezed orange juice
- 1 tablespoon chopped fresh rosemary
- ¼ cup granulated sugar

Core the pears and cut them into 8 wedges each. Arrange the wedges on dessert plates and drizzle with orange juice.

Combine the rosemary and sugar and sprinkle over the pears. Done-zo!

CITRUS SMOOTHIE BOWL

Makes 1 serving

I could have put this in the smoothie section, but it's so luscious that it had to be a dessert (the banana and avocado also make it a little thicker than your average suck-it-down smoothie). This bowl is vegan, gluten-free, raw, oil-free, refined sugar-free, soy-free . . . but full of fresh tropical flavors. It's also a dessert that's really good for you, between the hydrating coconut water and the vitamin boost from the spinach. Mix and match toppings; if you're thinking dessert, sweet additions like cocoa nibs and a little extra agave should do the trick. If you'd rather save it for breakfast, you might want more nuts and seeds for energy.

FOR THE SMOOTHIE BOWL:

- ¾ cup coconut water
- 1 cup fresh baby spinach
- 1 large frozen banana
- ¼ cup packed mashed avocado
- 1 teaspoon orange zest
- 1 tablespoon chia seeds
- 1 tablespoon flax seeds
- 1 tablespoon fresh lemon juice
- 2 ice cubes
- 1 to 2 teaspoons agave syrup, or more to taste

TOPPING IDEAS:

Granola
Flaked coconut
Golden raisins (just a few)
Blueberries
Dried pineapple bits
Pumpkin seeds
Cocoa nibs

Place all the smoothie ingredients in a high-powered blender and blend on high until smooth. Add a little more agave if you want to make it sweeter.

Pour into a bowl and add your favorite toppings. Get your spoon and enjoy every sweet, citrus-y bite!

INSTEAD OF:	USE:	BECAUSE:
1 cup white flour	⅞ cup whole wheat flour	More nutritious, more filling, more fiber!
1 cup whole wheat flour	¾ cup whole wheat flour, ¼ cup almond flour	Less gluten and a tiny hit of protein and omega-3s
1 cup granulated sugar	1 cup unsweetened applesauce (and reduce the amount of liquid in your recipe by ¼ cup)	Save hundreds of calories—like 670!
1 cup oil	½ cup oil, ½ cup unsweetened applesauce	Equally as tasty in muffins and sweet breads
1 cup canola oil	1 cup coconut oil or olive oil	Canola is low in saturated fat, but other oils give you more flavor
1 cup butter	1 cup mashed avocado	Better fat with more nutrients, still a great taste
1 cup butter or oil (baking)	1 cup mashed banana	Fewer calories and added potassium, fiber, and B6
1 cup cream	1 cup evaporated skim milk	Big drop in fat content
1 cup white rice	1 cup brown rice	More nutrients and fiber
1 whole egg	2 egg whites	Lower cholesterol, more protein
1 cup sour cream	1 cup Greek yogurt (the real stuff)	Half the fat and calories
1 cup sour cream	1 cup low-fat cottage cheese	Cuts the fat, boosts the protein
1 cup whole milk	1 cup skim milk	Fewer calories, less fat, same amount of protein—and lots of tasty ones out there

CHAPTER 7

MORE TIPS & TRICKS FOR GOOD MEAL-ING

Congrats! You own this whole healthy-eating thing! Morning, noon, and night, you know what to eat that will feel right for your body. At this point you should feel very comfortable in your kitchen, and you might even feel like you can call yourself . . . a cook. I hope you'll keep experimenting to figure out which foods you like to make and eat, and how they can improve the way your body feels. The tips and tools in this section are all about boosting your sense of empowerment. I've included a handy-dandy list of food substitutions, plus advice for what to eat when you're stuck in places or situations that aren't ideal for staying on track.

FOOD SUBSTITUTIONS

These are simple tweaks that will make your favorite recipes healthier and more power-packed. Try the substitutions on page 156.

WHAT TO EAT AT . . .

I know this all takes effort, but the effort should be starting to pay off. You're putting good stuff into your body, so you should be getting good stuff out of it. (I mean that literally: Your digestion and elimination should be spectacular if you're adding all this healthy fuel to your motor.) You should also have more energy, clearer skin/eyes, a more curious palate . . . and a sense of pride in taking care of yourself. But what happens when your good intentions go awry?

You're ready, willing, and able to partake in a salad bar, but the only thing you can find are fast-food restaurants. You're on a work trip and you can't get to a grocery store. Or a vending machine is your only option. Here are some solutions for when you can't eat what you ideally want to eat.

Here's what to eat at . . .

. . . a fast-food joint.

I'm not the biggest fast-food eater anymore, but I have to say, when you're in a bind, fast-food salads aren't all bad. These chains are really responding to consumers' desire for healthier choices. If you are like, "I must eat fries!" Then get fries—but get a small.

. . . a vending machine.

You've counted out your nickels and dimes, and you have just enough for a snack. Choose granola bars, fig bars, or protein bars if they're an option. Go for pretzels (as opposed to chips) if you crave salt. And if all else fails, choose peanut M&M's over plain—at least you can get a little protein!

. . . a birthday party.

Fruit! There's usually fruit at a birthday party. And if someone is pressuring you to eat cake, take it, say thank you, and ditch it when she (unfortunately, it's always a she) isn't looking. If it's an office birthday party, wait to arrive until you hear your coworkers start singing "Happy Birthday," run into the conference room, cheer for the candle blowing, and run back to your desk bluffing about an important e-mail you have to send out that MINUTE. If you're going to feel deprived, keep a bar of real dark chocolate in your desk and break off a little hunk as a treat.

. . . happy hour.

Happy hour is tricky because your defenses are down, treats/eats are cheap, and people are HAPPY. You can be happy, too! Walk into the HH knowing what you're going to order in advance (for example: "I'm up for one appetizer and one drink.") Try to avoid anything that's deep-fried (appetizer) or blended (drink). And remember, happy hour is generally a short window of time—so if it's not working for you, you can come late and split early.

. . . a gas station/convenience store.

Your friends wanted Slurpees, so now you're in the middle of the chip/candy/packaged sandwich aisle with a craving. Try an energy bar with the lowest amount of sugar in it. It's more filling than Fritos, and it should give you at least a little bit of nutrition.

. . . Starbucks.

I'm sure you know by now that all those amazing blended drinks taste super amazing because they are loaded with sugar. Listen, I know that sometimes you just need yourself a Red Velvet Cake Crème cappuccino . . . but you don't need the biggest one on the menu. The blood sugar dive your body is going to take when it's all over isn't worth it. Consider lighter options like an iced coffee or tea. And if you're hungry, you're in luck because Starbucks now has lots of healthy options. Their Protein Bistro Box is a winner.

. . . Dunkin' Donuts.

See above. Go for a real coffee or iced tea instead of a blended who-knows-what. And remember, just because the place has "Donuts" in the name doesn't mean you need to eat doughnuts while you're there. I will admit; as a former doughnut-aholic, I pretty much have to stay away from DD when I'm looking after my well-being.

. . . a frozen yogurt shop.

Again, I'm so not like, NEVER HAVE A TREAT. Just know that instant gratification can sometimes be overrated. Keep an eye on portion control at the places where you can serve yourself your own yogurt (filling up a third of one of those giant cups should be plenty). And when it comes to toppings, skip the candy bars and go for the fresh fruit.

. . . chain restaurants you find near malls.

It's not so bad to go to these joints once in a while! Many of them have "light" menu options. One of the perks of these places is that the prices are low and the portion sizes are huge—so consider sharing your meal with a friend to avoid "blargh" stomach as you're walking back out to the parking lot.

. . . a Mexican restaurant.

Dude, you can totally eat Mexican. Just go easy on the cheese, sour cream, and re-fried beans. A lot of Mexican places offer vegan options (especially in California), and I love to take them up on it.

. . . a sushi bar.

Pretty much anything goes at a sushi bar in terms of finding something relatively good for you. Just try to avoid things that are fried (tempura) and rolls that are made with mayo or cream cheese.

. . . the salad bar.

You're a real bar-hopper, aren't you? The big trick at a salad bar: Eat SALAD. Like, lettuce. And veggies. Don't go nuts on the premade pasta salads, tuna or potato salads, or basically any of the stuff that has a lot of mayonnaise or oil in it. Pro tip: Instead of going with a creamy, fat- and sugar-filled dressing, either go with oil and vinegar or see if there's a lighter pasta salad—like orzo and feta—that you could use in place of a dressing.

. . . an institutional cafeteria.

You're visiting a friend at the hospital or stopping by an office commissary, but you don't want to give in to the huge vat of mac and cheese. My choice is salad and a turkey burger without a bun: protein for energy and veggies to help me feel full.

. . . a vegetarian restaurant.

You should be able to feel good about ordering anything at a vegetarian restaurant, right? Sort of. You just want to avoid an all-carb meal. Make sure you get a protein in there from beans or legumes, and take it easy on the cheese, for the sake of digestion if not calories.

. . . the mall/food court.

I'm an adult, and I'm *still* entranced by the idea of getting to pick from all the different restaurants in a food court! Luckily, these days there are more and more healthy options. Look for Middle Eastern or Japanese places, since they tend to offer more vegetarian options and fewer cheese-filled or fried items. Otherwise, try to avoid meat on sticks, pizza, and fried rice.

. . . the airport.

So, so many snacks to eat at the airport! I'm generally too nervous about salmonella to eat something salad-ish or smoothie-ish at Terminal 2, so I say go with a protein bar, popcorn, or nuts. Note to self: Bring your own to save $$$. Check out page 55 for some of my favorite snack ideas.

. . . on an airplane.

I hear that once upon a time an airline gave you a meal of your very own, even in coach! Well, those days are pretty much over, probably for the better. Before I turned over my new leaf, I once brought pizza on a plane, and only as I opened it and, like, a dozen sets of passenger eyes locked on to me, did I realize that eating food with a strong aroma isn't the greatest choice in an enclosed space. (Plus, pizza.) Nowadays I bring a little bag of trail mix (see recipes on page 57) to get some protein in . . . in-flight.

. . . the movie theater.

See my unfortunate Sour Patch Kids story on page 18. Now I order a small popcorn, no butter, and a sparkling water or seltzer to avoid taking down a vat of diet pop. ENJOY THE SHOW!

WHAT TO EAT WHEN . . .

Above, I gave you tips on what to eat at places where your ideal food choices might be limited. But what do you do when you're stuck in a situation that's going to throw you off your game? Never fear—you will eat, and you will be okay.

Here's what to eat when . . .

. . . you left your lunch at home.

Here you made a nice salad for yourself, and it's still sitting in your fridge. That's fine; you'll eat it for dinner. But for lunch, don't give yourself license to go crazy. Try to approximate the lunch you planned to have rather than going off the deep end.

. . . you're having crazy cravings.

Crazy cravings can mean a few different things. For me, it's usually that I'm hitting the low blood sugar zone. If that's the case, I try to eat some of the snacks in my stash, like trail mix or rice cakes with almond butter. Then, once I'm feeling solid, I can get back to business. Another reason for cravings can be that you're feeling emotional. Try not to "feed the feelings," as they say. Reach out to a friend or distract yourself until the feeling passes. And if you're PMS-ing, well . . . God bless you; do what you have to do, within reason.

. . . you get home at nine, instead of six.

I'd recommend that you skip the big hearty meal you had planned for dinner and go with a smoothie instead. Or try a light breakfast for dinner. You don't want to go to bed on a full stomach.

. . . you just want to eat cereal.

Eat cereal. Just maybe not Lucky Charms.

. . . you're making dinner for your kids or staring at their leftovers.

Are you a mom who is suddenly on the chicken nugget diet? Sucks! They are so tasty, but aren't you so over it? A few things to try here: One is making your food BEFORE you make theirs, so you're not tempted to dine on pizza rolls. The other thing is to . . . and I know this is crazy . . . make your kids the same meal that you'll be eating yourself. If you know something isn't good for you, is it that good for your kids? Try making little forays into maturing their meals or eating something you'll all like (for example, the Spaghetti with Turkey Meatballs & Sauce on page 119).

. . . you're cooking. And noshing. And cooking. And noshing.

When I'm cooking, I end up grazing the whole time. So I'll put out *one* healthy snack to keep me company, like a bowl of grapes or baby carrots.

. . . you're cleaning up after dinner.

There's those last couple of sweet potato fries on the plate. The last piece of bread in the basket. Why let that food go to waste? People are starving! The only problem is . . . *you're* not starving. You are full. Save what you can for leftovers. And if you're feeling super guilty about the starving people—and yes, there are way too many people in the world with empty bellies—then "offset" your cleanup, just like you offset a carbon footprint, and make a donation to an organization like No Kid Hungry.

. . . you wake up famished in the middle of the night.

Are you *really* famished? Can you really not wait until morning? Then try to fill yourself up with a glass of water or almond milk—but no chowing in front of an open fridge.

. . . you're having dinner at your mother's/mother-in-law's.

Can you say trigger warning? A lot of us women have this thing with our mothers where they pay way too much attention to what we eat (or what we don't eat). Especially at our M-I-L's, we don't want to offend anyone, so we end up eating too much, or eating things we don't want, or eating stuff because it's just a habit, or revenge eating for some infraction that we never got over when we were thirteen. Guess what? You're not thirteen anymore. You're a grown-ass woman. You are in charge of what goes into your mouth. If anyone (MOM) is overobservant or offended, she'll get over it. Better let her get used to you making your choices now instead of decades of food drama down the road. Eat what you want, not too much, stop when you're full. Done-zo.

. . . you're at Thanksgiving/Christmas dinner.

See above. Also remember that, if you've recently become vegetarian or vegan and people are asking you dumb stuff like, "How can you have Thanksgiving without a turkey?" you don't have to defend your choices or engage in a discussion. Laugh it off. Or say, "That's a good question! It *is* different this year!" But they can eat what they want to eat, and you can eat what you want to eat. You could even bring your own dish so you know there's something you are going to enjoy eating while you're there. (May I suggest the easy-to-transport Baked Sweet Potato Fries on page 95, or the Savory Roasted Potatoes & Sprouts on page 100?) On the flip side, if you've been eating mostly vegetarian and you want some turkey or ham, go for it. The food police will not come to your house on Christmas Eve, or ever.

. . . you're about to exercise.

If you're planning on doing a big workout, a protein-carb combo will get you through it. When I'm strength training I like to feel full, but not so much if I'm doing cardio like running or spinning. I like to have real Greek yogurt and fruit, or apple slices or brown rice cakes with almond butter just before a little workout, but I'll eat 40 minutes to an hour before a big throw-down. Some favorite choices: quinoa or brown rice, half of a chicken wrap, or even a Lentil Veggie Burger patty (page 117). Don't forget to grab your reusable water bottle so that you can stay hydrated while you exercise. Instead of Gatorade (which can have a lot of sugar), try coconut water. It's super hydrating and full of potassium, which is great for just-worked muscles.

. . . you've just finished a workout.

After you exercise, your muscles need to rebuild. To make sure that you are re-pairing broken muscle fibers, you need to eat protein. Consider grilled chicken and vegetables with olive oil, a veggie omelet with avocado, or a tuna sandwich. Some No-Frills "Gourmet" Chicken (page 122) would also do the trick! Sadly, the myth that chocolate milk is the perfect recovery is just that—a myth.

. . . you want soup.

You can have soup! Just stay away from the canned stuff that is packed with so-dium! Try the tomato soup recipes on page 142 or Big Group Lentil Soup on page 139.

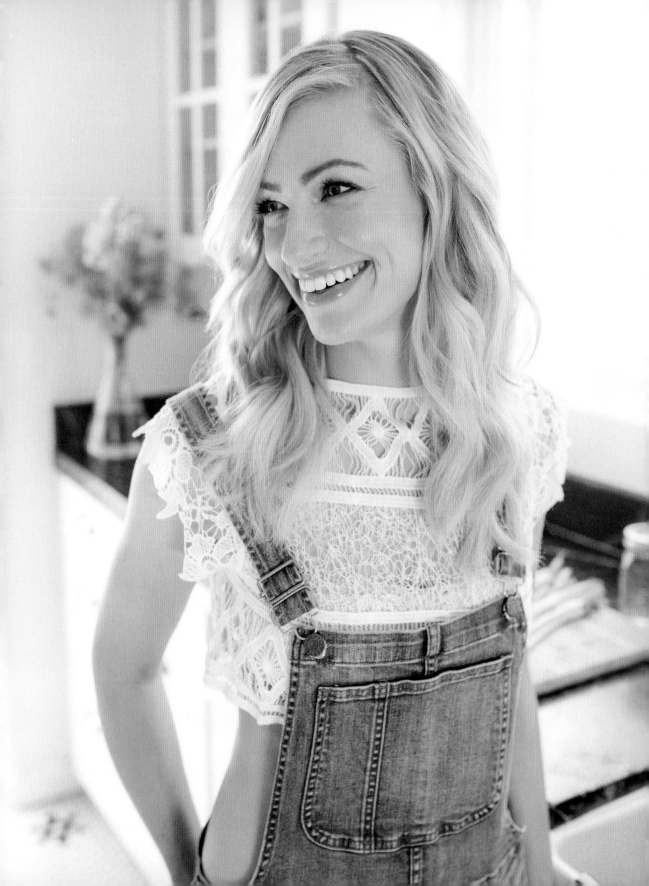

CHAPTER 8

BEAUTY FOODIE:
USING FOOD FOR BEAUTY AND WELLNESS

Earlier in this book (see page 60), I talked about "eating beautifully." That's because the food you eat can, not only make you feel beautiful, but also look more beautiful, too, from the inside out. But it turns out that food can also be a beauty tool to use on the *outside*. Using your kitchen to beautify your skin, hair, and nails provides alternatives to store-bought products and cosmetics that are, not only cheap and accessible, but also much cleaner than the kind you find at the department-store counter, which can be filled with toxic chemicals and additives. Here are some fun beauty hacks to try with foods that you'll find in your fridge or pantry.

BETH'S FAVORITE BEAUTY HACKS

Coconut Oil = Moisturizer and More!

Use coconut oil on your skin, and it'll feel as smooth as a baby's bottom—and smell like a piña colada. After an awesome vacation/bad episode of sunburn in Mexico, I was peeling and flaking all over my face. I tried two full nights of slathering with coconut oil. It cost me all of $5 and it worked like a charm. Besides being a fantastic moisturizer, coconut oil makes for a great hair protector before a dip in the ocean. You can use it as makeup remover when you're in a pinch—just smooth some over your eyelids and wipe clean with a cotton ball. You can also use it for "oil pulling," which is basically an Ayurvedic teeth-cleaning alternative to brushing that is said to remove harmful bacteria and naturally whiten your teeth. Swish some coconut oil in your mouth (it's helpful if you melt it first) for 15 to 20 minutes, spit it out (spit it into a trash can, not the sink, as solidified coconut oil can clog pipes), and rinse. Google "oil pulling" for more info.

Avocado = Face Mask

For a simple and cheap face mask (that's also fun to apply, especially with friends), mash half a very ripe avocado in a bowl, add about ¼ cup of honey, and apply to your face. Wipe it off after ten minutes. You should have nice, soft skin! Avocado and honey are both very moisturizing, and honey has antibacterial zit-killing properties.

Grapeseed Oil = Wrinkle Remover

Studies show that grapeseed oil contains antioxidants that may reduce damage to skin cells and improve your skin's elasticity. Try smoothing a little grapeseed oil on your skin to help reduce the appearance of wrinkles and stretch marks. You can also add a drop or two to your moisturizer to enhance its effectiveness.

Tea = Hair Shine Treatment

To give your hair some extra shine . . . try tea! Steep two teabags (golden chamomile for blondes, rooibos for redheads, black for brunettes) in two cups of boiling water for about ten minutes, then LET IT COOL. (Please, please let it cool.) When you take a shower, shampoo your hair, rinse, and then pour the tea over your hair, rubbing it into your scalp the same way you rub in shampoo. Leave it on for ten minutes, then wash and condition to maximize the gloss.

Orange Peel = Teeth Whitener

You can gently scrub your teeth with orange peel to get some whitening power. The citric acid on the outside of the peel breaks down plaque, and the spongy white part inside scrubs it away. Rinse with water and hold off on a full brushing with toothpaste for at least an hour.

Apple Cider Vinegar = Acne Treatment

If you're prone to acne, apply a little bit of apple cider vinegar to a cotton pad and gently use it to clean your skin after rinsing with water, then let it air-dry. It'll help tighten pores and kill bacteria. So what if you smell a teeny bit like salad dressing? Worth it.

Bananas = Shaving Lotion

You know bananas are good for your insides . . . but did you know that a bit of mashed banana can work as a shaving lotion as well? Mash it up, add a little water so it's not too thick, then go ahead and shave with a disposable razor. You'll end up with nice, smooth legs . . . but you may also crave a snack.

Plain Greek Yogurt = Skin Reliever

I can't stop raving about Greek yogurt . . . which can also be used as a healing tool. If you get a mild sunburn, apply a layer to your skin for a cooling effect. Just don't lick it off. Or do . . .

Eggs = Hair Conditioner

Use this neat egg conditioner about once a month: On clean, damp hair, apply ½ cup beaten eggs (both whites and yolks for normal hair, egg whites only for oily hair, and egg yolks only for dry hair). Leave it on for about twenty minutes, rinse with *cool* water so you don't end up with an omelet on your head, and then shampoo again.

HERBAL HEALING

To me, food isn't only about nutrition and digestion; I use lots of different foods and herbs to take care of my health. My family and friends call me "The Witch

Doctor" because I've turned into an herbal-remedy whore. I'm basically made of ginger and garlic now. I smell like a Chinese restaurant, but that's a good thing.

Okay, I admit it: I'm obsessive about my immune system and using natural remedies. I cannot play Caroline Channing on *2 Broke Girls* and flip into dumpsters and jump off walls and get stuck in windows unless I'm 100 percent healthy. Plus, I love using things around the house to make me feel better when I've got a cough or a cold.

Herbal healing isn't just ideal for day-to-day stuff—it can make a big difference for people who suffer from chronic diseases. My mom has lupus. Under supervision from her doctor, she changed her diet to avoid inflammatory foods like sugar and white flour while increasing consumption of anti-inflammatory foods like fruits, vegetables, and whole grains, and it's worked wonders.

I suggest you try eating or drinking some of my go-tos below, and see if they help you:

Add Coconut Oil to Your Tea

Not just a beauty tool. It's a natural antiviral—Kat Dennings taught me that one! It also supports your metabolism's fat-burning capabilities.

Drink Chlorophyll Water

Chlorophyll gives plants energy and is found in green, leafy vegetables. I add drops to my water—it tastes like nothing—and find that I get a real energy boost. A bottle is about $10 and lasts for a long time. I make sure I have a glass of it every single day, especially on set when I need some extra energy.

Toss in Chia Seeds

I like to put chia seeds in my smoothies. I soak them overnight and then throw them into my Vitamix with the other ingredients. Organic chia seeds give you energy, and they're a good source of fiber, too. They also have plenty of omega-3s that improve brain function—so I add chia seeds to everything when I'm learning dialogue for the show.

Sparkle Your Water (No Sugar Added)

It's sooo tempting to grab a Coke, but sparkling water quenches my fizz needs without 39 grams of sugar and food coloring! As I mentioned in the section about water (see page 53), my favorite brand is LaCroix. Zephyrhills and Poland Spring also have nice sparkling waters . . . and there's always a classic sparkling mineral water like Pellegrino. When I'm not feeling fizzy, Mountain Valley spring water is my go-to. It tastes like I'm drinking from a stream in heaven (seriously), which makes it worth a little bit of extra $.

Get a Wake-Up Call

Every day at work, I order the same get-me-going drink: water, lemon, ginger, and cayenne. You can make it yourself with warm water, juice from half a lemon, an inch of grated ginger, and a dash of cayenne pepper. It heats up my body and gets my whole digestive tract moving!

Bone Up on Broth

You've probably been hearing about bone broth lately—a food/beverage that people are catching on to, including the LA Lakers, who have made it a staple of the team diet. You can simmer your own bone broth, or buy it in a jar at the store. I like to cook rice in it for flavor and an immunity boost when I'm feeling oogy. Word on the street is that the collagen in the bones can enhance the collagen in your skin, giving you a brighter appearance.

Revel in Lavender Oil

In addition to its great smell, lavender oil has powerful aroma-therapeutic qualities that ease stress and aid relaxation. I take a whiff or dab it on my scent points when I am feeling panicky or anxious. It also happens to be a natural sanitizer; search "lavender oil hand sanitizer" online for lots of easy DIY recipes.

Melanie, a good friend of mine and a fellow actress, is super obsessed with her immune system, just like I am. Pretty much the first thing we talk about when we see each other is the newest herbal remedy we use to stay healthy. She taught me this disgusting yet useful tip: When you start to notice the first signs of feeling run-down or like you're getting sick, eat a piece of whole wheat or gluten-free toast with a few cloves of crushed garlic on top (garlic has antibacterial and antiviral properties that have been shown to control infection in the body). NOTE: It'll burn like a mother#$%$%$! Don't use too much—one time I did two slices of bread with like six cloves, and I immediately threw up. BUT, every time I've done this right at the beginning of getting sick, I've knocked the virus out before it started. Talk about a ME-tox!

Here are some other edible/drinkable ways I fend off colds—my very own "health crack":

- Inhale steam with garlic cloves. Fill a pot with water and a few cloves of garlic. After it boils, put a towel over your head and the pot and breathe in that steam. When I do this, Michael doesn't know if I'm sick or if it's dinnertime.
- Eat spinach like WHOA! Popeye it up! Pound it like crazy when you feel under the weather. You can eat it straight up or add it to your smoothies, sandwiches, omelets . . .
- Go for absolutely ZERO sugar. (I know this is a super-hard one—but it really makes a difference if you cut out all sugar the moment you feel like you're getting sick.)
- Drink chlorophyll water. (See above! Kat and I swear by it!)
- Have hot water with lemon every morning—it's amazing for hydration and your immune system.
- Make my wake-up-call drink mentioned above: warm water or tea with lemon, cut up chunks of fresh ginger, and a dash of cayenne pepper.
- Add cinnamon and raw honey to hot water—they're antiviral!
- Take turmeric, zinc, vitamin D, and garlic supplements, and of course drink Turmeric Tea (page 52).
- Down green tea—it's full of amino acids called L-theanine that relieve stress and anxiety.
- Buy oregano oil from Whole Foods or a health-food store. It works wonders in fighting colds and also gives you an energy boost.

Part II

MOVE YOUR BODY

EVOLVING FROM SUPER SLUDGE TO MAJOR MOVER

So I made it through my first season on the show, and I was excited to start the second. I was also eating like a champ, and everything was better because of it. My skin was glowing, my eyes were clear, my sleep was better, and my digestion was like . . . whoa! For my season-two checkup, I went back to the same doc who had previously told me I was vitamin deficient, assuming I was going to get a gold medal. She checked me out, sat me down, and told me, "Beth, you have to exercise."

What? Where's my trophy? And seriously . . . *another* thing for me to do?

It's not that I mind moving my body. Actually, I really like to wiggle it (just a little bit). Sports were always a huge part of my life. I was a major athlete from the time I was four or five—T-ball, b-ball, soccer . . . basically, all the balls. (That's what she said.) At fifteen, I was playing on my eighth-grade soccer team *and* junior varsity, as well as a travel soccer team, so my body was pretty much always in shape. I had a giant Mia Hamm poster on my wall. Plus, my family was always very active. We took bike rides, hung out in parks, and went for walks. My parents were both runners, and my younger sister, Emily, and I were lucky to have them as fitness role models. My dad, Dave, explained that this didn't happen by accident: "When my brother and I were adopted from an orphanage in

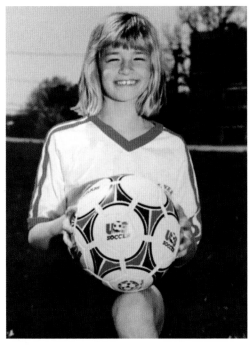

Age 10. Most embarrassing soccer photo ever.

Oklahoma City, my adoptive parents couldn't walk us for more than a few feet without us getting tired. They were diligent about getting us involved in sports and exercise at an early age to keep us healthy." Now, keeping physically fit is just part of his lifestyle. Even in his midfifties, my dad is running, weight training, cycling, and walking—and he even tried yoga. (His favorite pose? According to him, the "double down dog.") All this exercise, coupled with a heart-healthy diet, has led to a better quality of life. Even on holidays, we all eat . . . and then we go on a family run. Dave means business!

In college, my performance program was super physical. I was required to take ballet, jazz, and tai chi (a gentle, flowing form of martial arts) as part of my acting training. When I think of the number of times we were doing calm, meditative tai chi under the morning-light-dappled trees on our luscious green campus . . . and then running to puke in the garbage can . . . oh boy. We can blame the $1 bottles of André "Champagne" for that. Let's just say I wasn't super healthy when I was doing those workouts.

When I finished school, I was up to *here* with bills, working three jobs, and sharing a one-bedroom apartment with no money for gas, let alone workout classes. My health and my weight started to suffer. My metabolism definitely slowed down. When I was in this "no money, no time, Easy Mac–eating" phase, I really let the athletic part of my life go.

As you know, when I booked *2 Broke Girls*, I threw everything I had into work. I ate, slept, drank, and poo'd Caroline Channing. It was all I could do that first season to go from food junkie to nutrition buff. So the doctor's new order to capital "E" exercise felt like yet another task, something else I had to deal with on top of work, press, photo shoots, and trying to make time for family, friends, and my boyfriend. Like so many of us, I didn't think I had room for another "to-do" in my life. But the doctor was right the first time, so I had to figure out a way to make working out work for me.

As with eating well, I knew I'd have to put an exercise regime on a slow burn, like, so slow that Axl Rose would release that rumored solo album before I could really start working out like a champion. Indeed, it did take a long time before exercise and movement felt like a welcome element in my day. Then the "task" started to feel worth it when I noticed the change that initially came from gentle movement and yoga. It was a SLOW progression. Snail slow. Turtle slow. Oscars on a boring night slow. But sure enough, my energy level began to increase and my head began to clear. It was like a fog was lifting. I felt more alert and adept at my very physical job, and stronger in general. I wasn't looking for a six-pack or the ability to win a marathon—I wanted and needed a renewed sense of self and connection to my body. And I got it.

Don't think of exercise as a "task" anymore; think of it as ME-TOX TIME, which is a much better motivator. It's a moment in your day when you can solely be focused on getting stronger while jamming out to great tunes or an interesting podcast and loving your body. It's not about how it makes you look on the outside (though fewer butt dimples is a plus FOR SURE) . . . but rather, how wonderful you feel on the inside.

What worked for me was making an initial commitment to myself to "kinda, sorta" exercise, and I'd recommend the same plan for you. Each day I choose the type of exercise I'll do and the duration based on my mood. If I'm feeling stressed out and overwhelmed I do yoga at home, sometimes with the help of an app. If I'm feeling angry and annoyed by some conflict or drama with work or relationships, I do cardio, like running or paddling, taking a spin class or getting on an elliptical. If I'm tired, I go for a walk or a hike—every time I get outdoors I feel better. The fresh air and vitamin D revive me. You just have to gauge how you're feeling and what your body is capable of doing. You ideally want your workout to make you feel empowered, strong, and happy, whether it's a sweaty gym session or Zen bliss in the yoga studio. Lemme tell ya, there are still days when the thought of going to the gym makes me want to drive off a cliff. But then I think about the upsides: the surge of energy and strength, the cardiovascular improvement, my growing body confidence. It's a much healthier boost than some of the other things I used to do when I needed a quick fix.

WHEN I NEEDED ENERGY, I USED TO . . .

Pound sugar. Sugar gives you a burst of energy, right? You think you'll have a Coke and a smile. Well, if you've ever seen a kid eat a candy bar, run around like crazy, then crash hard, you'll understand why sugar is a childish solution to a grown-up problem. When you eat a sweet treat, your level of blood sugar spikes, giving you an energy boost . . . that is incredibly short-lived. Suddenly your blood sugar drops, leaving you feeling tired and lethargic (and usually craving more sugar). If you're really craving something sweet, a piece of fruit is a better choice because it usually has some fiber along with its natural sugars, which will slow down the blood sugar roller coaster in your system.

Down caffeine. Same issue as above. You may get a quick energy boost from that cup of java or soda, but it will fade as quickly as it arrives. The caffeine stays in your system for hours and could affect your ability to sleep when it's the right time (leading to a vicious cycle of feeling worn-out). One way to modify a coffee boost is to add milk to your late-afternoon latte. Milk has protein in it that your body can convert into energy.

Take a nap. Taking a nap is actually a good option when you are fading. For some people, twenty minutes can do the trick; others need an hour to get real restful results. But you can't just pass out at your desk (unless your coworkers are like, "Whatev"). A workout can take the same amount of time, burn calories, and give you a much bigger energy boost.

Chug an energy drink or snack on an energy bar. No solution here . . . just the sugar and caffeine issues from above. By the way, most "energy" bars have the same ingredients (and sugar content) as a candy bar.

Pick a fight. Well, that wasn't exactly standard operating procedure for me, but anger and stress can boost your energy by causing adrenaline to course through your system. The problem is that, after the adrenaline rush wears off, you crash. And someone's pissed at you.

Snort a line. Kidding. Never did that.

HERE'S HOW YOU START: BIT BY BIT

Once you decide to get your body moving, you'll need a strategy. Here's a two-week plan to kick off an exercise habit that will make it feel like a WANT as well as a MUST:

DAY ONE: Take a ten-minute walk. No need to strap on your exercise bra or special gear—just get out there, move, and breathe. (Experts say that going from zippo to ten minutes a day can significantly improve heart strength and general fitness!)

DAY TWO: Take three minutes to stretch out a little bit before you begin your walk. Nothing Bendy Barbie–worthy, just stuff like bending down and touching your toes, then rolling your back up real slow before you stand tall again. Twist from side to side. Tilt your head from left to right, and back again. Now trot.

DAY THREE: Add two more minutes to your walk. So, stretch for three, walk for twelve. That's just fifteen minutes out of your day—nothing you couldn't sneak in during your lunch break, before going to work, or while walking out to your car to go home for the day. Continue this for the rest of the week (and if you feel like you want to add some walk time, go for it).

DAY EIGHT: Try something new. A yoga class, perhaps? Even online in the comfort of your own home? (See page 197 for suggestions on where you can find classes online.) I'll fill you in on the physiological and mental benefits of yoga on page 212, but for now I can tell you why yoga is my go-to choice. You don't have to feel intimidated by yoga—you can go at your own speed. While I recommend learning the ropes in a beginner's class, a solo practice is ultimately as fulfilling to do at home on your own. Your focus will be on balance and flexibility, paying attention and listening to the natural resistance and acceptance in your body. Give it a try. If you're still hesitant to downward dog, consider a dance or swim class.

DAY NINE: **Go back to your walk.** Twenty minutes total, plus stretching . . . and you might want to stretch again as a cooldown.

DAY TEN: **Try your yoga/dance/swim class again!**

DAY ELEVEN: **Walk again.** Twenty-two minutes of walking total, plus stretching. Then add a few ab crunches at the end (see page 193).

DAY TWELVE: **Try something that feels like play instead of exercise.** Swimming, tennis, biking, dancing, hiking with a friend . . . pick one and stick with it for at least 30 minutes.

DAY THIRTEEN: **Bring your walk up to twenty-five minutes, plus stretching, and repeat the ab exercise that you did the day before yesterday.** Now add a resistance- or strength-training suggestion from page 188.

DAY FOURTEEN: **Stick with the usual.** Stretch. Walk (or do your cardio of choice) for 30 minutes. Finish with your ab exercises plus one other resistance- or strength-training exercise. Stretch again as a cooldown.

You officially have a routine! It generally takes about two weeks to form a new habit, and you've formed the best one you possibly could have for your long-term wellness. Congrats! For good cardiovascular health, you want to get to the point where you're exercising at least thirty minutes a day, most days of the week. Once you're in the flow you'll feel like thirty minutes is way too short, but that's all you need to aim for if you're short on time.

WHAT'S YOUR WHY?

Ask yourself: What's motivating me? Weight loss is a pretty common motivator, but as we talked about earlier, it's not the only reason to exercise. There's building strength, relieving stress, calming anxiety, boosting energy, and just generally improving your health (there are very few chronic health conditions that aren't bettered by getting moving). I know why I had to start moving my body . . . I was sick way too often. My period stopped. My energy was flagging. The doctor suspected that my adrenal glands weren't functioning correctly and knew that exercise could help alleviate all of these symptoms. She was right.

Maybe you just like the stretchy clothes, the pop of color in the shoes, or the cute guy/gal who works at the juice bar in the gym.

All of these are legit reasons to start working out or increasing the exercise that you already do.

Just remember, how are you going to start? Small.

Just as I did with changing the way I ate, I had to make small shifts in order to change the way I moved. I'll suggest three levels for you to try: start with LITTLE SOMETHINGS (also known as Meh Workouts), increase to BIGGER BREATHS (which I fondly call "Cardio, Schmardio"), and then invite your pals to join you in some GROUP MOVES.

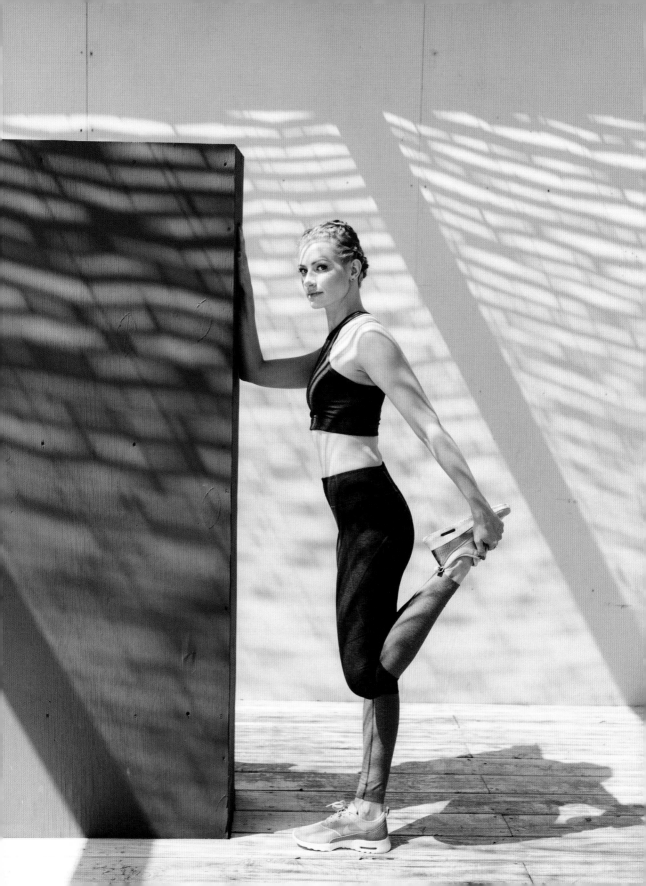

CHAPTER 9

LITTLE SOMETHINGS
(A.K.A. MEH WORKOUTS)

A little something is better than a lot of nothing. If you don't feel like doing a full workout today, then tell yourself, "I'm just going to walk around the block, or do ten minutes of sun salutations, or some combination of breathing and movement." It's what I call a "Meh Workout." Just ten minutes of breathing and stretching will ease your muscles, increase oxygenation in your body, improve your concentration, and even relieve stress or anxiety. That's a whole lot better than doing nothing.

The best thing about a Meh Workout is that it can happen anywhere, even when you're chilling out on the sofa. Don't be confused: "meh" doesn't mean the movement doesn't matter, it just means you're not strapping yourself into Spandex and paying a gym membership to make it happen.

Beth, I like what you're saying here.
Cool!
You look really great, and it sounds like you feel really good, too.
That's super nice of you.
But I just can't do this.
I've heard this somewhere before. Try me. Now.

I CAN'T EXERCISE 'CAUSE . . .

I don't have time.

No one has time. We really don't. So think about exercise in advance and put it on your schedule just like an appointment or a meeting. Keep the appointment with yourself just like you would with someone else.

I'm so tired from work.

Of course you are. Work is exhausting. But this is going to *increase* your energy. Tell yourself that you're just going to do ten minutes of exercise. Just ten minutes, that's all you need. I bet once you're in it and you're starting to sweat, you'll end up doing more.

I have a headache.

Getting your blood pumping may actually help you get rid of that headache.

I just ate.

Why don't you wait for twenty minutes, just like you had to do when you were a kid and you wanted to get in the pool right after you ate a hot dog and potato chips? Use those twenty minutes to plan your workout or figure out your exercise schedule for the upcoming week.

I'm not feeling well . . . I think I'm getting a cold.

You know what's great for fighting off colds? Exercise. If your lungs are really compromised, I understand taking the day off, but if you're just talking about a stuffy nose or a sore throat, you should move ahead with movement. The breathing you'll do while walking or jogging can act as a natural decongestant. Yoga or breathing exercises could also help raise your immunity to whatever's invading your system. Just stay away from anything too strenuous when you're really under the weather; your body needs to rest.

I'm bored of my routine.

That's because routines are boring! Let's change it up today! Crank up your favorite motivating music and create a little cross-training circuit with a bunch of different exercises. See page 187 for tons of exercises that you can choose from.

The class is full.

Well, that's a great excuse! I'm going to suggest that the exercise gods stepped in today and decided they didn't want you in that class anyway. You're already in your workout wear, though, so let's take a power walk or run #likeagirl instead. If you're at the gym, try a type of cardio that you've never done before.

I just feel really self-conscious.

Everyone feels self-conscious before they start a workout regimen. The good news: No one is paying attention to you. Stop worrying about what everyone else is thinking and focus on what you're thinking instead, which should be along the lines of, *I want to do what's right for my body.*

I don't have the right equipment.

You don't need equipment. Just your body. See page 192 for details.

My trainer got sick.

Look at you with a trainer! Hopefully your trainer has shown you the ropes, so you can proceed without him or her around. At the very least, you can do a little bit of cardio on a treadmill or an elliptical machine.

All my workout clothes are dirty; I should do my laundry instead.

Been there, done that. But guess what—you're just going to stink up your clothes again, so give them a squeeze of Febreze, slide on that nasty exercise bra, and go for it. Or wear clothes that aren't your "exercise" clothes, like a T-shirt and a pair of shorts. What's happening *under* the clothes is way more important.

I can't afford fancy workout gear.

While there's something to be said for getting fully Nike'd up, I still make it burn in my old soccer shorts, exercise bra, and Forever 21 workout clothes. What you're doing inside is so much more important than what you're wearing outside. If you can't spend big bucks on Lululemon pants, no biggie. Maybe throwing down $10 for a headband/wristband set or cool water bottle will motivate you.

My muscles are sore; I can't bear to do more work right now.

Fair enough. If you've had major workouts two days in a row, then it's a good idea to give yourself a day of recovery. You know what's great for recovery? Ten minutes of stretching.

It's too hot out.

No sweat. Maybe you don't do that nine-mile run, but what about swimming instead? Or something indoors? Just be sure to stay hydrated.

It's too cold out.

You do have to be careful exercising outdoors when it's super cold outside, but look at skiers and snowboarders—they're having lots of fun in chilly weather! Make sure you've got the right protective gear on, including sunglasses and sunscreen if the sun is reflecting off snow. Or head indoors to do what you gotta do . . . even if it's just skipping rope.

I'm pregnant.

Mazel tov! What a great time to exercise and keep your body strong and healthy for yourself and your baby. And while you don't have to be one of those women who runs a marathon the day before she delivers (yes, they exist), you should make exercise a regular part of your pre-baby routine.

I'm stuck at home with the kids.

Okay, a few thoughts here. First of all, look at page 187 to get ideas about working out at home and even creating your own "home gym." Second, use the kids as part of your workout—if you're dealing with babies or toddlers, you can actually use them instead of weights. Finally, remember that kids love to play. So play with them. Run around with them. Play tag, hide-and-seek. Not only will you be raising your heart rate and increasing your strength, your kids will see you as a role model: a mom who likes to move.

It's too early in the morning to work out.

Keep in mind that your workout will wake you up even more efficiently than hitting snooze on your alarm clock or chugging your venti black. And then you'll be DONE and off to an excellent start, with the whole day in front of you.

It's too late at night to work out.

Working out isn't only energizing, it can also help you get a great night's sleep. Instead of cardio or strength training, consider restorative yoga, deep breathing, or stretching instead.

It's dark outside/it's not safe.

You've found a good excuse not to exercise. Please don't go for runs late at night or in neighborhoods you don't know. Just not worth it. Luckily there are lots of exercises you can do right at home, or in your hotel room if you're on the road. (Note: I'm not a huge fan of working out alone in hotel gyms either.) See page 187 for loads of ideas.

I'm too lonely.

Oh, you need a workout buddy! A workout buddy is someone who can keep you company, keep you accountable, and keep things interesting. Ask a friend to join you for a walk or a hike, or to sign up for the bike next to yours at spin class. Or do something that requires two people, like playing tennis or kayaking. You'll be having so much fun that you won't even realize you're exercising.

I hate the showering part.

Hmm. I don't know what to tell you there.

Listen, I get it. We know exercise is good for us. We know it's what we have to do to live long and prosper, so to speak . . . yet we are so resistant to making changes that will improve our lives! So here's the question of the day-slash-lifetime: If we know all these things, then why don't we automatically do it? My answer: It's all about instant gratification. You work out once and expect to walk out of the gym looking like Serena Williams. Not going to happen. It takes time, and it takes consistency. You have to stick with it for a while to see results. But instead of waiting for that six-pack for motivation, keep track of all your results, like decreased blood pressure or better-fitting pants. Every little bit helps. And also remember that action is the key to change. Nothing can change if you don't do something about it. Exercise is action, and it will change your body and your life for the better.

My bestie Matt Doyle believes this 100 percent. In addition to being a wildly talented actor and singer, he's also a personal trainer. Matty and I met at auditions for *The Sound of Music* when he was fourteen and I was fifteen. We auditioned together to play the teen lovers Liesl and Rolf. Matt won the role of Rolf, but a different girl booked Liesl. He came up to me at the first rehearsal, gushing, "I just don't understand how you didn't get Liesl. I loved your audition. You were *perfect*." I looked at him and said, "It's all good—I'm Maria!" We love to look back on this and laugh. From that rehearsal on, we were inseparable. We even went to prom together. Matt ate dinner at my house every Sunday evening with my family. He was part of my family then, and fifteen years later, he's still my family. Here's how and why he got into fitness:

Growing up, Beth was always active. She was very athletic and constantly pushing herself from a young age. Watching her score on the soccer field or take over the dance floor, I was always inspired by her energy and positivity.

When I moved to New York City to become an actor, the directors and producers I worked with encouraged me to get into shape. Initially, I welcomed fitness into my life purely for vanity reasons. But as I became more active, I discovered the same energy and positivity that Beth had always possessed. I got hooked. The effect that fitness has on my mind alone is enough to keep me going back to the gym. Like Beth, I struggle with an anxiety disorder. I'm amazed by how much an active lifestyle helps to control my anxiety. It keeps me focused, driven, and happier in general.

Fitness became such a positive influence on my life that I decided to become a certified personal trainer. Now, I am fortunate to teach at Barry's Bootcamp in New York City, passing that positivity on to my clients. I love having Beth in my classes and getting the opportunity to work out with her (and even push her beyond her boundaries a little bit). Even when we go on vacation, we both make it a point to do something fun and physical together, whether it's kayaking in Austin or going for a run along the Pacific in Seattle. It's amazing to have my closest friend by my side, motivating me to live an active and healthy lifestyle.

Matty! Thanks so much! You totally inspire *me*!

HOME SWEET HOME: WORKING OUT WITHOUT LEAVING YOUR HOUSE

In order to start an exercise regimen, there's no need to invest in a lot of fancy equipment or pay for an expensive gym/club membership. You can do everything you need to strengthen your body within the privacy and comfort of your home. Here's a list of my essential home-gym gear that you can use in all kinds of ways, without spending a lot of $$$. (Shopping hint: Search Craigslist, sports consignment shops, or Amazon for cheap buys.) I'll give you some of my favorite moves that use these items, and you can also do a quick search online to get tons of good ideas.

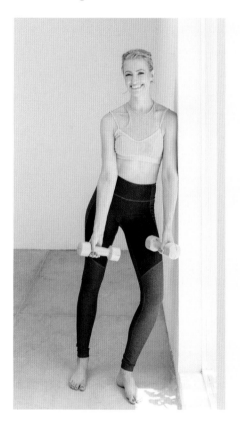

Definites

Dumbbells. Great for arm, shoulder, and chest exercises. I recommend having two sets: a lighter set (for me, five-pounders) and an eight- to ten-pound set. That way you can build up strength, while still using the lighter weights for extra pumping power when you walk or run.

DUMBBELL EXERCISE:
Classic Overhead Press

Stand with your feet hip-distance apart, knees soft, and arms shaped like a football goal post. Using the lighter set, extend your arms straight over your head, then lower them back down to goal posts. Start with twenty reps and work up to more.

Resistance bands. These are particularly useful when you're tight on space, and especially when you're traveling—just throw them in your bag! Like the dumbbells, I recommend getting two—one lighter resistance and one heavier resistance.

RESISTANCE BAND EXERCISE: Seated Crisscross Row

Sit on the floor with your legs stretched long and your knees slightly bent. Wrap the band around the soles of your feet and hold each end of the band with the opposite hand so that it makes an "X" shape. With your palms facing the floor and your core nice and firm, pretend you're rowing a boat. Slowly pull your elbows back so your hands come to your waist, then slowly extend your arms long. Repeat for two to three sets of twelve reps.

Medicine ball. Fun fact: It's called a medicine ball because it's so good for your health. These soft, weighted balls have been around forever . . . even gladiators used them! Now you know why Russell Crowe looked fiiiiine . . . I particularly like using a medicine ball for core and arm strengthening. They come in a lot of different weights, but I like a ten- to twelve-pounder.

MEDICINE BALL EXERCISE: Wall Ball

Holding the ball in both hands, put your back against the wall and squat down so it feels like you're about to sit in a chair. Hold the squat and lift the medicine ball above your head. Hold it there for 30 seconds, then release and do it again. Try to do three in a row without coming out of the squat.

Jump rope. Nine zillion kids can't be wrong. Great for cardio in a pinch.

Extremely Useful

BOSU ball (depending on your budget). A BOSU ball is one of those dome-shaped contraptions you've probably seen at the gym—it's hard and flat on one side and soft like a ball on the top. When you do strength-training exercises on it ball-side down, like squats or push-ups, you're working your core and also all those little muscles that help stabilize your entire body.

BOSU BALL EXERCISE: One-Legged Bridge

This will strengthen your core, glutes, and hamstrings: Lie on your back with your right foot on the dome of the BOSU ball. Extend your left leg up to the ceiling at about a 45-degree angle. Keep your arms on the floor at your side, palms facing up. Pressing your right foot into the dome and keeping your core tight, lift your hips until your torso is even with your right thigh. Really use those hamstrings and glutes! Hold for two beats, then lower yourself down to your starting position. Repeat fifteen times, then switch sides.

Stability ball. These big, round, bouncy balls are really great for core work, especially if you have lower-back issues. And they're also perfect for total-body strengthening. (Note: They're also really fun to bounce on when you have friends over.) The only downside is that they can take up a lot of room, which is the only reason I didn't include one in the "definites" category.

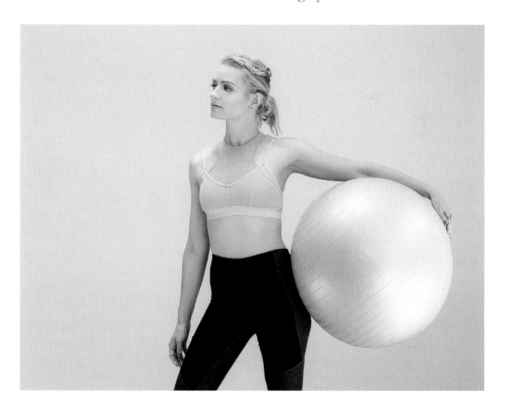

STABILITY BALL EXERCISE: Reverse Crunch

Lie on the floor on your back with your arms at your sides, palms facing down. Rest your heels and lower calves on the top of the ball. Exhale and bring your knees in toward your hips until your feet are resting flat on the ball. Keeping your hips up, hold the position for a few beats and then inhale as you stretch your legs out again. Repeat ten to twelve times.

Yoga or exercise mat. I love my yoga mat for preventing slips and slides while I'm doing yoga or floor work. It also helps me create a dedicated space when I'm working out. But you could also skip the mat and use a few beach towels instead (as long as you're on a carpeted floor; it would get too slippery on a hard surface).

Foam roller. Roll your body over this lightweight cylinder at the end of your workout to release tight muscles and prevent stiffness the next day.

Splurges

TRX. A TRX Home Suspension Trainer is super easy to set up (you can just pop it over a door), and it's really portable, too. (The army ships them overseas for soldiers to use to stay fit—so what's your excuse for not working out on your next business trip?) It basically lets you do a full strength-training routine using your own body weight. And there are lots of videos online offering differing workouts, so you can always change things up. It will run you about $200, but I think Santa would like to bring it to you next Christmas.

TRX EXERCISE: TRX Squat Jump

Holding the handles of the TRX down and a few inches in front of your waist, step back until you feel the tension in the straps. Bending your elbows to keep the straps where they are, squat down. Then push your arms down so you feel the resistance in your triceps . . . and jump up! When you land, find your squatting position and do it again. Aim for ten reps.

Gliding discs. These small discs let you glide over any surface (wood floors, carpeting), so you can do full-body toning while challenging your stability. All that sliding around gives your workout a new dimension because it makes your body work in new dimensions. The discs are small, portable, and versatile. Helpful hint: Do not try to move heavy furniture with these gliders. That's a completely different infomercial.

GLIDING DISC EXERCISE: Glider Slide Lunge

Stand with a foot on each glider and your arms next to your body. Slide your left foot out about double hip-width to the side, bending your right knee, until you are in a lunge position. Bend your elbows to 90 degrees with your hands in front of your chest, like you're holding imaginary cross-country skiing poles. Return to starting position and lunge again, on the same side. Repeat twelve times, then switch to the other side.

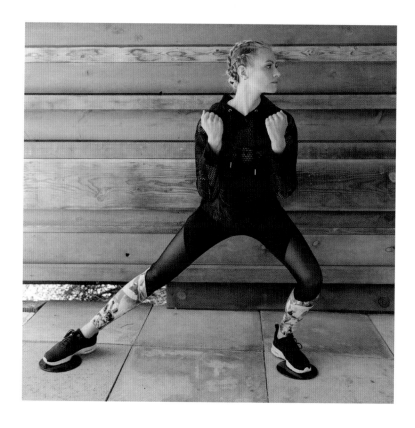

Mini-trampoline. You'd be stunned at all the different ways you can use a mini-trampoline—and that it's actually a great workout. Turn on some tunes and jump, jog, run in place, kick . . . your heart will soon be racing. Look on YouTube for routines you can follow. Plus, it's easy on the knees for anyone who needs to give those joints a little TLC.

MINI-TRAMPOLINE WORKOUT:
Five-Minute Trampoline Workout

Minute 1: Keeping your feet in the middle of the trampoline, bounce to warm up.

Minute 2: Jog on the trampoline, starting with your knees low and then bringing them higher and higher toward your chest.

Minute 3: Jumping jacks! Start with just the arm movement, and once you get used to it, get your legs involved.

Minute 4: March! Try to bring your knees up high enough so that they're even with your hands. You can twist and march to work your abdominals.

Minute 5: Bounce again and try to even out your breath. Gently step off the trampoline when you're done—you're going to feel like you're still bouncing.

Portable speakers. Music really motivates me when I work out. It's fine to have headphones blasting in my ears, but there's something about cranking up the beats so the whole house reverberates that really keeps me going. I'm a big fan of the Jawbone Mini Jambox, but any portable speaker will do. Check out page 219 for my favorite workout jams.

NO-EQUIPMENT-NEEDED MOVES

You don't need a home gym (or even to be at home) to bust out these moves. You can do them in any order, at any time, for as long as you wish. Build a whole workout around them, or just sneak one or two in whenever you have the time.

Jumping Jacks: Great for revving up your heart. Get to it for one minute, just like you're at camp. Or military school.

Plank on Wall: A fantastic way to engage abdominal muscles, especially for post-pregnancy moms. Lie belly-down on the floor with your feet touching the wall and your hands lined up under your shoulders. Press up to plank position, then walk your feet up the wall until your body is parallel to the floor. Hold for one minute. Rest for thirty seconds. Then repeat.

Elbow Plank with Opposite Arm Reach: Another genius core exercise. Push up into a plank position on your forearms. Stretch your left hand in front of you and reach to the right. Breathe while you hold the position for one minute. Repeat on the other side.

Wall Jump Squats: These strengthen all the muscles in your legs and help build bone density while you're at it. Face the wall and squat deeply (like super deep, y'all). Jump, lightly touching the wall as high as you can with both hands. Immediately reset and repeat. Try to do this for a minute and a half, building up to getting in at least thirty reps.

Frog Crunch: This move gives you nice, strong abs while helping you open up and strengthen your hip flexors. Lie on your back and bring the soles of your feet together. Bring your knees up to your midline as you lift your shoulders, traditional crunch–style. You'll look like a frog on her back. Do a set of thirty. Rest. Repeat.

Burpees: Burpees work almost every muscle in your body. They're like sun salutations that really kick your butt—but they're so worth it! Start by standing up straight, then bring your body down to a squat as you place your hands flat on the floor in front of you. Kick your legs out behind you into a plank position, drop down and do a push-up, then hop your legs back in so you're once again in a squat. Jump up and clap—you've got nineteen more!

Donkey Kick Pulses: These are genius for your legs, lower back, core, and butt. They can put a little pressure on your knees, so you might want to do them on a mat or a towel. Get down on all fours, with your hands below your shoulders and your knees even with your hips. Tighten your abs. Keeping your knee bent, lift your left leg behind you so the sole of your foot is parallel with the ceiling. Using your glutes and hamstring, pulse your leg thirty times. Lower your leg and repeat on the other side.

Half Banana Abs: Another excellent exercise for your core. Start flat on your back with your arms reaching up to the ceiling. Beginning with your chest, roll up while lifting your left leg, and reach for it. Lower back down and repeat with the right leg. Aim for twenty reps, alternating sides.

Mountain Climbers: These build lower-body and core strength, while also getting your heart pumping. Start in plank position with your hands beneath your shoulders. Bring your right knee into your chest, return to plank position, then repeat with the left knee. Right, left. Speed up the switch. It's going to feel like you're running in plank position. Do it for at least one minute.

Walkouts: Another winner for core strength, in addition to upper-body strengthening. Start by standing with your feet hip-width apart, then bend over and place your hands on the floor. Shift your weight onto your hands and walk them forward until you're in plank position. Keep that core strong! Walk your hands back to the original position on the floor. Repeat for a set of ten.

Push-Ups: Old-school. Classic. The key is to keep your back and abs nice and strong. Do them on your knees if the traditional toe version is too tough. Go for a set of ten.

Triceps Push-Ups: As you may have guessed, this is your key tricep workout. Triceps push-ups are a little easier than classic push-ups, so you have to do more! Sit on the edge of a chair, ottoman, or coffee table and rest the heels of your hands just next to your hips. Press into your hands and lower yourself to the floor, then push back up again. Come on, I know you can do a set of twenty!

Plank Leg Lifts/Dips: Core city. In plank position (clearly my favorite) with your hands or elbows on the floor, lift your left leg, then bring it down and under your body for a dip. Swing it back out to starting lift position. Now switch to the right leg. Do ten on each side, alternating legs.

Jumping Lunges: Sooo perfect for strengthening your legs. Stand in a lunge position with your left foot in front. Jump, switching your legs midair so you land in a lunge with the right foot in front. Do this as many times as you can in a minute. You will feel like a superhero.

Chair Squats: These are great for your quads, hamstrings, and butt. Stand in front of a chair and slowly lower yourself down as if you're going to sit. Then, using your core and not your arms, lift yourself back up into a standing position. (PS: Not to get too graphic, but you can practice this exercise using the toilet as your chair as well.) Do as many as you can in one minute.

Chair Push-Ups: To balance out the chair squats and work your upper body, do push-ups using the chair rather than the floor as your starting position (but do not do this with your toilet). Face the chair and put your hands on the edge of the seat, with your body at an angle. Do as many push-ups as you can in one minute.

Cooldown: Stretch. Take a deep breath. Curl up into child's pose. You're all done.

LIVING ROOM WORKOUTS

If you don't want to create a workout space in your home, then your couch will do just fine. Hell, you can even make it burn (mildly to super hot) while you watch your favorite shows. I do some of my best Meh Workouts at home in my living room, usually while I'm watching TV. If I'm feeling super lazy, I'll just lower myself up and down from the couch using my triceps (see Triceps Push-Ups above), or I'll hold on to the side of my couch with bands on my ankles and do leg lifts. But if you can force yourself to get up off your butt, try the following:

Scandal Squats
(Feel free to reward yourself with red wine, Olivia Pope–style)

As you watch Kerry Washington and the Gladiators "handle it," slowly do ten to twelve squats in a row. This not only works your legs but you'll also feel it in your core.

Bachelor Bands
(With or without wine)

Tie one of your bands around your ankles and one around your knees. Every time a bachelorette cries, slowly try to spread your legs apart and bring them back together. Or, if you want to do something standing, slowly squat down into chair pose, then slowly come back up. Amazing for your legs and booty.

Mob Wives Medicine Ball
(Don't drink and ball!)

While the Mob Wives (or Real Housewives!) go after each other, lift your medicine ball over your head and then slowly lower it down to the floor, bending into a deep squat. Your shoulders and booty will say "Thank you!"

Big Bang Theory Ballet Bod Bonanza

When some of the Victoria's Secret angels appeared on *2 Broke Girls*, Kat and I asked them about their workout secrets. They swore by this instructional DVD that they do on the go called Ballet Beautiful. It was developed by this amazing ballerina named Mary Helen Bowers (the very same ballerina who helped Natalie Portman get her plié on for *Black Swan*), and it shows how to do the same exercises that dancers use to get long, lean, and toned. I figured if almost EVERY SINGLE Victoria's Secret angel swears by it, it must be genius. And once I checked it out, I was sold. Now I always bring either the DVD (or her even-cheaper book) with me when I travel. It's an amazing workout you can do anywhere, especially if you're working your abs AND laughing at Jim Parsons. Your arms and booty will be tight as Jane Fonda's circa 1982. I'm still praying these moves will make me more graceful so that maybe my pratfalls will be calculated instead of by accident. But this workout is definitely making me more flexible—which translates to less icing and Epsom-salting when I come home from a super-physical day on set.

BOSU Basketball Playoffs

As a sports fan, I always feel more inspired to work out while watching world-class athletes I admire do their thing. Also, there's some major eye candy among those athletes. LeBron? Federer, anyone? I even get a little weak in the knees watching Carli Lloyd. Cheer for your favorite team while holding a squat on your BOSU ball for two to three minutes at every basket—or goal, or touchdown. No BOSU? That's cool—you can still squat without one.

Game of Thrones Gut Buster

Hold a plank position for at least a minute anytime you see blood. Follow with twenty medicine ball crunches when someone sleeps with one of their relatives.

*Walking Dead*lifts (modified)

A deadlift is that exercise you see hard-core weightlifters do where they raise massive dumbbells up to their chests while their muscles bulge and their veins explode and you think their eyeballs will pop out. Fitting for a zombie show, right? What you're going to do is take a light-weight dumbbell and stand it on its foot. (If you don't have weights, use a two-liter bottle of water or something that weighs at least a couple of pounds.) Every time a zombie gets killed, you bust this move: Keeping your back straight at a 45-degree angle, squat down and grab the head of the dumbbell. Tighten your abs and lift the dumbbell by standing up straight. Do ten reps per zombie walker.

MORE MINI-WORKOUTS
(AND THEY'RE PRACTICALLY FREE!)

Retro YouTube Videos: The treasure trove of workout videos on YouTube are free, hilarious, and amazing. You have to check out "8-Minute Abs/8-Minute

Buns"—such a throwback! And be sure to look up exercise videos from the '80s; I do these before bed, and I swear they're just as good as a Pilates class.

Ten-Minute Yoga Routines: These are all over the Internet, and there are tons of apps (Yome is a good place to start). You can also look for free yoga routines on sites like Do Yoga with Me, Be More Yogic, and Yoga with Adriene.

Jump Roping/Hula Hooping: Fun, cheap, and easy to do while binge-watching *Breaking Bad* on Netflix.

Shadowboxing: It's harder than you think. Throw punches and jabs while keeping your feet moving for three minutes at a time, with a thirty-second rest period in between. It's a perfect stress-reliever if you imagine being in combat with your boss/landlord/ex . . .

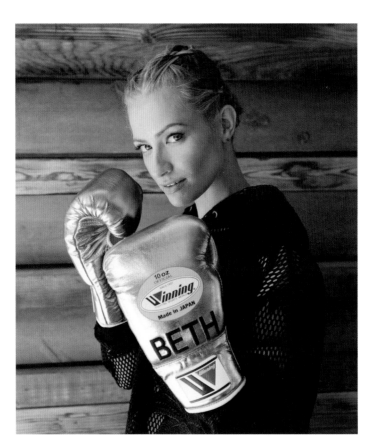

PPSB: Push-ups, planks, squats, bicycle crunches. Get to it.

Stair-Down (and Up): Try climbing your stairs at home ten times in a row. Your quads will burn, burn, burn. In a good way.

Fun with Balls (not that kind, sicko): Kick, hit, or throw a ball around for ten minutes. It's super fun and your heart rate will zoom up.

Lunch Break Lifts: If you have a twenty-minute break at work, you can do a little workout. I keep a set of resistance bands in my dressing room. The writers on the show have them, too, along with yoga mats and foam rollers for doing some stretches when they can. Even my dad will do a workout at his desk or take a quick twenty-minute run to clear his head for the second half of the day. He has the option to stop in to the school gym and take a shower, but if your refreshment options are limited, you can always pat down with some deodorant and baby wipes if you get your glow on.

WHOA, GIRL

If intense aerobic exercise is causing you major stress or pain, dial it down. Take deep breaths, stretch, and go for a gentle jaunt around the block instead.

At this point your house might be looking like one big gym to you—and that's a good thing. Find little opportunities to get movement into your life all over your house and throughout your day. Little things like making your bed and washing dishes by hand instead of putting them in the dishwasher (or leaving them in the sink . . .) add up as tiny, consistent energy boosters that make your body function well and dose you with the feel-goods. And they'll make you feel more and more entitled to move out of the "Meh" zone and into the fun, body-boosting world of true-blue cardiovascular exercise.

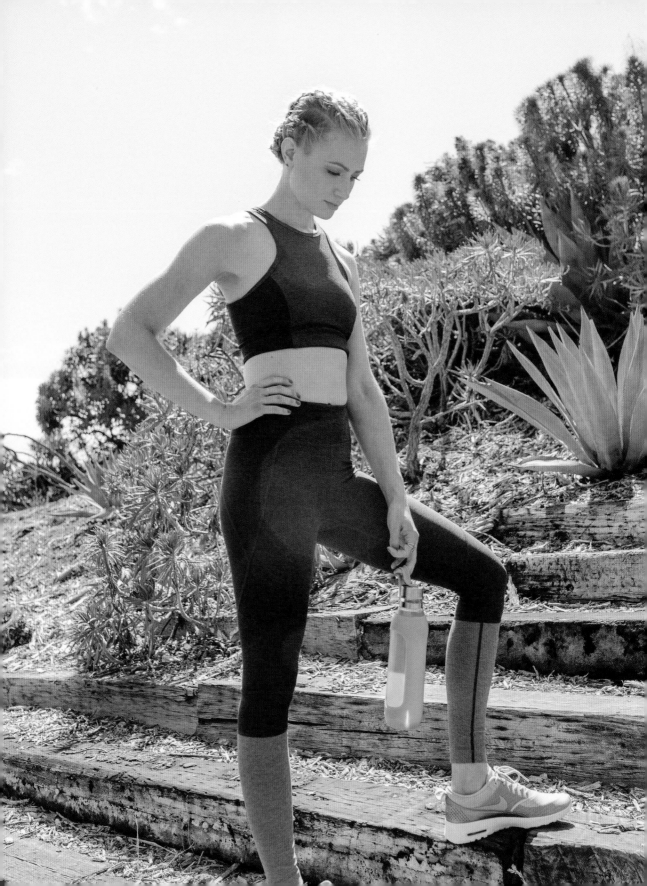

CHAPTER 10

BIGGER BREATHS
(A.K.A. CARDIO, SCHMARDIO)

In the previous chapter, we talked about lots of easy, cheap ways to bring a little bit of exercise into your life. Whatever your motivation, you've hopefully found ways to take small steps that have prepped your mind and body to take it to the next level. That next level involves taking bigger breaths and requires more strength and energy—in other words, "Cardio, Schmardio."

You'd have to live under a rock to not know that exercise is good for you, with noted benefits for your cardiovascular health and immune system. Many people like to work out to build strength, flexibility, and coordination, or to lose weight. But the benefits of exercise are bigger than just fitness. Exercise can also:

Relieve stress
Combat depression
Help you sleep better
Cure hangovers
Improve your mood, concentration, memory, and ability to learn
Make you feel happier (by raising endorphin levels)
Raise confidence and self-esteem
Elevate your sex life

Oh, I'm sorry . . . you don't want any of those things? Then you are not human, my friend. We all want and need at least a few of the things on this list,

201

so add them to your private list of "Reasons I'm Moving My Ass Today." On these pages you'll find lots of good ideas for fun stuff you can do, plus ways to keep yourself motivated.

I know that I have to change up my fitness routine all the time so that I don't get bored. When I have time and really want to get my heart pumping, I'll run, speed-walk, hike, bike, and swim. Anything to stay out of the gym if I can.

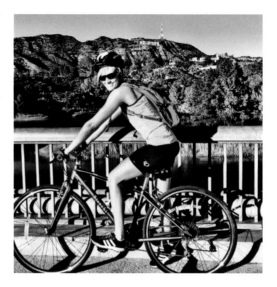

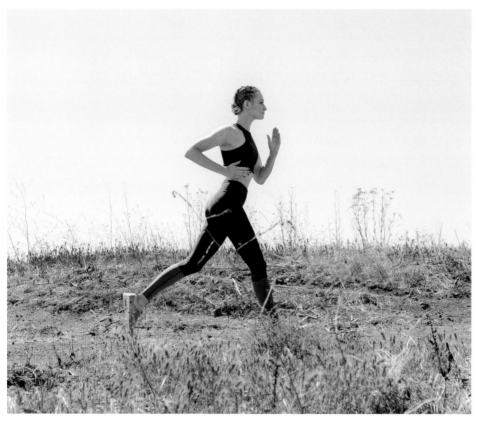

Wow, it looks like I'm running really fast. Or maybe not. I can't tell.

Then there's boxing, which I kind of LOVE. I found a boxing trainer at a no-frills boxing gym where I am one of the only girls who gets in the ring. I get dirty and sweaty and ugly and so into it. Newsflash: Nobody gives two shits. I can't stand girls who wear makeup and fake eyelashes to the gym. I tried to do a fancy gym for a while, and I lasted a month. I would rather be around sweaty dudes who don't care. I don't have a lot of time to make working out happen, and I'm not going to talk myself out of going because I can't put on a cute gym outfit.

Getting my Rocky on motivates me. But I understand how hard it is to stay motivated, especially when you're working out on your own. If weight loss is your primary goal, it might be more helpful to explore a class situation, or work with a trainer to keep you going when you want to stop. People love spin classes for that reason, too. Sometimes it really helps to have someone shouting at you and getting you to move. I grew up playing super-competitive soccer. I had a coach named Mort, who was so tiny—all of five feet tall and super skinny—but he was terrifying in conditioning. I guess you could say he scared me into action, which worked for me at the time. My dad was a motivator, too, putting me through treadmill work-outs that kept me competitive as a teen. Some days, I still crave that. It depends on your personality; tough love might not be ideal for you. For example, Michael works out alone. He hates classes, and he has an all-or-nothing personality. He'll either walk, or he'll sprint 100 percent of the time, during his workout.

There are a few other ways to keep yourself motivated. One of them is giving yourself daily bursts of get-to-it . . . a little oomph each day. For example, I'll hunt around and read a book or a blog post related to my goal. When I was trying to improve my tennis game and get ready for matches, I made a Pinterest board of my favorite tennis players and tennis fashion from blogs. I also read *The Inner Game of Tennis* each night before bed (which helped me not only with my game but every other aspect of my life; I highly recommend it). There are tons of scripted tennis movies you can view, like *Match Point* and *Wimbledon* (a teenage fave of mine—don't judge), and documentaries up the wazoo. I highly recom-mend watching *Venus and Serena*, which will make you want to not walk but *run* onto the court.

When your motivation flags, try to connect your workout to causes you feel passionate about. For example, the only thing that kept me motivated to train for a half marathon was my intention to use it to raise tons of money for one of my favorite organizations, The Rape Foundation. Knowing that my running contributed to helping hundreds of victims of sexual assault made it a lot easier to wake up for training at 6 a.m. If running for a cause ain't your thing, organize a local basketball, tennis, or softball tournament with your friends and raise money for something that moves you. Or talk to your local gym about doing a friendly competition or mixer for a cause.

When all else fails, make your workout a competition. Find someone to best. As we've discussed, I'm super-duper competitive. And I'm a terribly sore loser. So when there's a time or a person I want to beat, I have a goal that keeps me motivated. Go ahead and make a bet with some friends and compete against each other to achieve your fitness goals . . . and the winner gets a (healthy) dinner, some cool workout clothes/gear, or to make it rain! With money. Not rain.

BETH'S MINI-MOTIVATORS: EXERCISE

Here are a few of my favorite ways to keep my brain occupied so my body can do the work:

You Can't Stop the Beat. Music. It's what keeps me going when I'm after those big breaths. I love anything Jay Z or Beyoncé . . . randomly enough, Mumford & Sons keeps me motivated . . . and Taylor Swift's *1989* actually made me enjoy running. I'd put that on and goooo! And I never got sick of T-Swizzle. I couldn't do more than three miles, but when I listened to that album I could distance run. Even right this minute, I can't help but think of this . . . sick . . . beat.

Power Playlist. Instead of listening to a full album, build a strategically planned playlist that features power songs around the hardest times of your workout (for me, that's the beginning and the end, right before cooldown). Check out page 219 for the songs that get me in mood.

Rousing Reads. Ah, the magic of audiobooks. There's nothing like having someone reading to you from an amazing book to keep your mind off what your body is doing. When I was training for a 10K, I lost myself in Amy Poehler's hilarious book *Yes Please*. Either of Mindy Kaling's books will do the trick, or get lost in the mystery of *The Girl on the Train*.

Podcasts. Another great motivator when you're walking or running a bit of distance. My favorites include the *Nerdist Podcast* and *WTF with Marc Maron* (I love interviews with comedians). I listen to NPR podcasts for some insight on what's going on in the world, and I feel like I get smarter when I tune in to *Radiolab* and *TED Talks* podcasts.

Stick, Meet Carrot. Promise yourself a post-exercise snack that you ONLY allow yourself to enjoy after you've completed a significant workout. You don't want to unravel the benefits of your session by going crazy with salt or sugar, but let yourself muse over the delicious taste of a filling smoothie or a scoop of sweet trail mix when you're all done . . .

Binge-Watch. Is there a series you've been longing to catch up on? Tell yourself you're only allowed to watch it while you're working out (that's how I fell in love with *The Affair*).

Envy. Simple. Work out with someone who is more fit than you.

Words to Win By. Stick a photo or quote in your gym locker or bag that REALLY means something to you. Look at it when you feel like you don't want to work out, and let it inspire you. One of mine comes from the movie *A League of Their Own*, when manager Jimmy Dugan (Tom Hanks) tries to rally the Rockford Peaches: "It's supposed to be hard. If it wasn't hard, everyone would do it. The hard . . . is what makes it great."

Stick to a Schedule. I've found that making an exercise journal or calendar helps motivate me and keep me on a schedule. I know that if I don't put a workout on the calendar, I'm not going to wake up on time. Now, every week I know what days to get up early, so I get it done. You can find super-cute schedule layouts online, and then add pics and quotes to get you going. (Check out Pinterest for even more ideas.)

ROCK YOUR BODY

One of the biggest objections people make about exercising is that they don't look the part. They're too fat. Too gangly. Too uncoordinated. But I believe that every body deserves to be treated well and worked out. You don't have to be pro athlete draft-ready to reap the benefits of moving your body.

You've got to understand that everyone has their issues, from supermodels to senators, and you just have to embrace yourself and your body for what they are. You have to enjoy your life and try to be healthy. More days than not I can tell myself that I like and appreciate the total package, and I think that's a respectful level of self-acceptance. Hey, I could try to be perfect . . . but I'd rather be honest with you.

My struggle is with my underbutt. Not my butt, but my underbutt, that chunk between the butt and the legs. Sadly, I don't have Kardashi-ass. No matter how healthy I eat and how hard I work out, it's still there. And while I pride myself on keeping my skin really healthy, I'm the first (and often the only) one to notice little red bumps that crop up for no reason. And then there's the lower belly area that almost every woman hates on . . .

Here I am, being so critical, and then one of my girlfriends goes and gets a nose job. I'm like, "What? Why do you need a nose job?" She looks great. I don't even notice noses. But you notice what bothers you, even if no one else does.

So I'm trying to shift the paradigm, so to speak. Instead of thinking, "I hate my underbutt," I think of it as, "Hmm, my muscles down there are really weak. That's not good for my legs and hips, and it doesn't help me when I'm wearing big heels for work. So what can I do to GET STRONG?" Not get beautiful, but get *strong*.

Changing negative thoughts—mine and others'—is a mission I've been on since high school. In middle school I had tiny chicken legs. It was just my body type at the time—I was athletic and I couldn't keep up the calorie count to stay juicy. I remember getting up the courage to ask out this guy I had a crush on, Kevin, and he responded with, "I'm not going out with you, you're anorexic!" That still stings all these years later.

When my family moved to the Bay Area, I wasn't as active. And I started to notice changes in my body. It wasn't that I gained weight per se, but there was a shift. I was a little girl with muscle . . . and that was over. Puberty hit and I got hips, and a butt. My negative-A-cup training bra filled out to a full A-cup. Major.

In Marin, the whole lifestyle is about health and the outdoors—bike riding and hiking to the beach. I liked being around that and wanted to encourage others to enjoy it, too, especially girls my age who seemed to be struggling with body image issues. So my friend Brianna and I led a body-positivity group where we'd discuss our body image and how to enhance it. During our free study-hall period, a bunch of girls would sit around a big conference table and do "check-ins" with each other. We didn't have to talk about our bodies . . . it was more like a girls' club where we could debrief and occasionally try out body image exercises and games that made us feel stronger. It was like body image book club.

Ironically, I've picked a career where my looks are constantly being evaluated, and that's a bummer. I was never, ever into makeup, but now I have to be done up all the time, whether it's for shooting or going to events. If I go easy on the makeup and go to business meetings, I often see my colleagues' faces kind of crunch up like they're thinking, "She doesn't look like this on TV!" It makes me feel insecure. A couple of years ago I went to the Tony Awards feeling like a million bucks . . . and looking like it, too. I was Spanxed from head to toe, but who cares? I was so smoothed out that I ate penne arrabiata before the show. But the headline the next day? "Beth Behrs' Wardrobe Malfunction!" Someone had taken a shot of me seated—and you could see the bottom hem of the Spanx peeking out from under my dress.

It was hardly world-shaking news, but gossip sites zeroed in on it. I shouldn't have given a rat's ass, but I couldn't help myself. So I surrounded myself with people who gave me lots of love and support.

Bottom line: My self-esteem still takes hits now and then. Like when a director gives me an offhand comment like, "Can you try to cry prettier?" (I have a legendarily ugly cry.) Or, "Beth, try not to scrunch your face so much." I'm like, "That's just my *face*." I try to let it roll off me. In those moments I just have to embrace who I am. And if I'm not cranking at 100 percent body positivity, then I get a spray tan and wear a sarong so my underbutt doesn't see the light of day.

The key for getting through those rough days is to turn your thinking around. Instead of criticizing yourself, flip it and think of three great things about yourself. Are you a good cook? Are you funny? Are you a good mom/wife/sister/daughter? Find things to love about yourself and be grateful for. Full self-appreciation is always going to be a day-to-day struggle, but you have tools you can use to offset negativity. Train your mind to see positives instead of negatives. So on those bad days, ask yourself what you love and value about yourself and how you can treat yourself with kindness and respect. You don't have to adore your body, but you can give it nutrition. You can move it. You can make investments in your body now that will pay off for a lifetime. You can rearrange your thinking.

So if you're telling yourself you can't exercise because you're embarrassed, or you're wondering, "Is everyone laughing at me?" . . . the short answer is: No. Nobody gives a shit. No one is looking at your body as critically as you are. Everyone is worried about themselves. You're a grown-ass woman and you can handle it. Now stop screwing around and start stretching out.

BODY TYPE HYPE

I want you to think about your "problem" area like I think about my underbutt: It's not ugly; it's not bad; it just needs a little love. So if you feel shame/angst/drama about _____ (fill in body part here), here's how you can make it good and strong. You're going to be exercising anyway, so think of your "problem" as part of the bigger solution. Be aware that "spot-training" (focusing on one specific area of the body) isn't some kind of miracle turn-around. You can do curls till you die and still not have Serena's biceps . . . though you will have stronger arms. You're not fixing, you're not correcting, you're just giving certain areas of your body a little extra attention. Embracing instead of ignoring. Discussing instead of dissing. Learning to appreciate your body for things like its strength or flexibility instead of rejecting it for some arbitrary aesthetic reason. Your body is special. It is singular. It is yours. So own every little bit of it. And if some part bugs you, here's how you can work on it:

My big booty bugs me.
First of all, understand that BB (big booty-ness) is super on trend right now. But if you want to make your butt muscles stronger and tighter, try a Side-Lying Leg Lift. Lie on your side with your legs extended out straight. Your lower arm can rest under your head; your top arm can rest on your hip. Lift the top leg up while keeping your hips steady and facing forward (do not rotate backward). Lower down and repeat. Aim for twelve to fifteen reps on each side.

My big boobs bother me.

Again, the grass is always greener. So many small-chested girls would trade you for your big rack! Well, let's just say that women with big boobs might want to avoid yoga inversions—but they might love the weightless freedom they feel swimming laps in the pool! If you've got large breasts and you want to tighten and lift your chest, try a Y-Raise (this isn't like a "we must, we must, we must increase our bust" move; it strengthens back and shoulders to help your posture). Using a pair of light dumbbells, stand tall with your feet hip-width apart, slightly bending your knees, and hold the weights in front of your thighs. Brace your core and draw your shoulder blades down and back as you lift the weights above your head in a Y shape. Then slowly return to your start position. Work your way up to four sets of twenty reps.

My flat chest flusters me.

Okay, smaller-breasted girls, it's your turn. To give your boobs a little extra perk, try Chair Dips. Sit down on a chair. Place your palms at the edge of the seat and point your fingers toward your feet. Shift your weight onto your hands and then walk yourself forward until your butt clears the front of the seat. De-hunch your shoulders and bend your elbows to a 90-degree angle. Now, lower your tush until your shoulders line up with your elbows, then press into your palms and push back up to where you began. Aim for two sets of ten reps.

My big muscles mystify me.

Oh, see, everyone wants big muscles, and here you are thinking you look too bulky. Fine, Muscle Mama. If you're looking to lean down overall bulk, try Pilates. It strengthens your core and tones muscles all over your body. And because it helps your posture, you'll have the appearance of looking leaner.

My skinny legs leave me lukewarm.

To make skinny legs stronger, walk around in high heels all day like I do. Not! Try squats, which not only strengthen your legs but also your butt and your whole body. Stand with your feet hip-width apart and keep your arms at your sides. Lower your body back as far as possible by pushing back your hips and bending your knees. Bring your arms out in front of you for balance. Keep your spine neutral and your chest lifted, and don't let your knees go out in front of your toes. Go down as far as you can, then slowly lift your body back up. Feel the burn! Aim for thirty reps.

My batwings bum me out.

You and everyone else. Your skin is your skin and it's going to do what it's going to do. But if you want to keep your upper arms nice and strong—not RIPPED, but strong, and add some strength to those triceps, try the classic Bent-Over Row. Grab a pair of small weights (or two water bottles). Lean forward and bend your knees, keeping your back flat. Extend your arms until they're straight. Squeeze your shoulder blades together, your back still flat and your elbows in and pointed up. Slowly lower the weights/bottles back to your original position. Go for two to three sets of ten to twelve reps.

My tallness troubles me.

Your days of shrinking down and hunching over are over. You're not only going to embrace your height and the advantages that come with it but you're also going to make yourself look even taller. That means walking with your shoulders back and your back straight. It also means walking proudly in high heels. Here's how you do it, according to shoe expert Meghan Cleary, author of *Shoe Are You?*® (shoeareyou.com) and designer of the shoe line MeghanSAYS:

> Walking in high heels is just like Pilates. Both strengthen your core muscles and guide you to pay attention to the middle part of your body, where all movements have their start.
>
> To begin, put your high heels on! Situate yourself in front of a full-length mirror, standing a few feet back. Look at yourself admiringly. Your legs are long, your calves voluptuous. Revel in your womanly glory. Next, close your eyes and mentally identify your core muscles and pelvic floor, your abs and transverse abdominis. Open your eyes and touch the muscles lightly with your fingertips so you can intrinsically intuit them. Take a big breath in and hold. Because your feet are no longer balancing you, your core is the place that will now need to keep you steady. This is the place you need to walk from. You will want to picture your legs scissoring out from this, your all-powerful core.
>
> (*Tip:* Do Tree Pose at least twice a day. This is an excellent yoga balancing pose that will give you more control as you speed through your day in stilettos.)

Now, take one step out with your right leg. Watch yourself in the mirror, observing how your leg relates to your core. When you feel steady on your right leg, put all your weight on that leg and pull up through your core for balance. Yes! You've got it! Now, gently bring your left leg forward past your right. See? Not so hard. Notice in the mirror how your body sways. What parts of you move and what don't? How do you look while moving your legs? Keep going and slowly move around the room away from the mirror, concentrating on your core and intending elegance in your moves. Try this at least once a day for fifteen minutes until you begin to feel steady. Then, hit the sidewalk to practice some more. Remember, even if you carry your flats in your bag and wear your stilettos only from the house to the car—know that you have succeeded!

(*Tip:* Envision that a string is running through the center of your body, from the top of your head down to your toes, when you are walking. It's a lot like ballet without the tutu.)

Tune in to your core, the most feminine part of you, be okay with teetering a bit your first few times out, and be willing to step out of your comfort zone. These are principles to guide you whether you are walking in stilettos or just zooming through life.

Thank you, Miss Meghan!

My shortness is a strain.
Follow Miss Meghan's advice above!

My flabby belly flusters me.
There are only two ways to get a perfect six-pack: work out several hours a day, several days a week, or get Photoshopped. Every woman worries that her belly isn't strong enough. But stop thinking about it as jiggle, and start envisioning it as the potential for core strength that will improve your overall health, posture, and well-being. You can go crazy with Pilates or ballet barre, but why not start with a classic plank? Hold the position for at least a couple of minutes a day—one minute in the morning and one at night. You can also try forty to fifty bicycle crunches to tighten your tummy from top to bottom.

My saddlebags stress me out.

If you'd like to strengthen the outside of your thighs and hips, try Traveling Squats with Resistance Band. Tie the band around your ankles and stand with your feet hip-width apart. Step your left foot out to the side as far as you can, and feel the resistance from the band. Then put your weight on your right foot and lift your left leg out to the side as high as you can (it may not be super high!). Keep your torso upright and try to point your toes slightly downward. Now, try it on the other side. Do twelve to fifteen reps on each side.

My general lack of coordination is a conundrum.

There's no spot-exercise to improve coordination, but there are lots of general workouts you can do. What I'd suggest for you and your potential spaz-ability is a dance class. You can try ballet if you really want to focus your movement, or something like Zumba, hip-hop, or salsa so you can let it all go!

YOGA

My absolute favorite form of Big Breath exercise is yoga. You're actually going to read this and be like, "All right, Beth, we get it, you LOOOOOOVE yoga." And that's okay because I'm a huge fan of yoga for everyone. There's a bunch of things I'll recommend for great cardio in the following pages, but yoga is by far and away my favorite. I really credit it for getting me on the right track in my life. Studies show that it reduces the risk of heart disease, lowers blood pressure, cuts cholesterol, and lowers BMI—and those are just the physical benefits. Anyone who practices regularly will tell you that it brings a sense of calm into their lives (including me). I have a friend, Sarah, who suffers from severe performance anxiety. She's incredibly talented but still has panic attacks when she's about to sing. She's been able to use yogic breathing to calm herself down before she gets onstage!

I have another friend who drinks four Diet Cokes a day, and I convinced her to try yoga. My little sister, Emily, is doing it as a sort of meditative thing to help her figure out what she's going to do after college. I got my mom, Maureen, to start yoga to help alleviate her lupus symptoms. Now she does it two to three times a week, and it's helped her so much. She's a real yoga success story (she likes to stay at the beginner level even though she can clearly move up). I got a friend who was trying to lose weight to do it. Even Michael likes restorative yoga, which involves

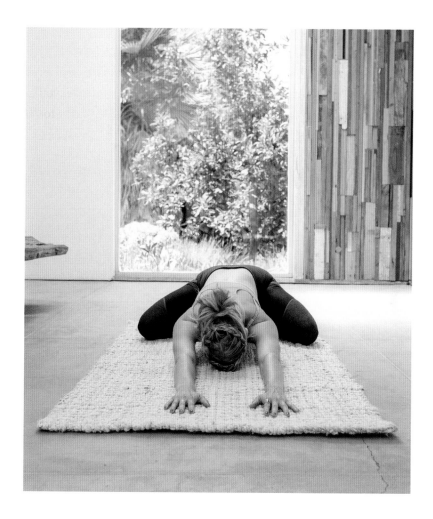

a lot of stretching and resting. He calls it "old people yoga," but maybe those old people are on to something!

Some friends of mine have said that they were resistant to try yoga because they didn't have a "yoga body." They felt too out of shape or too big. Jessamyn Stanley, a strong, curvy woman who has a series called "EveryBody Yoga," has talked about this problem:

Even with all the obvious benefits, there are still a million reasons people feel like yoga just "isn't for them." The root of many of those issues comes from the fact that the only widely recognized "yoga body" is that of a thin, affluent white woman.

And who can blame people for thinking that? This is the only type of person yoga companies, studios, and sometimes even teachers put any active effort in to attracting to the practice. This is a shame, because the eight-limbed path of yoga knows no size; it is completely unrelated to the lame beauty ideals that are heralded by the media and society at large. Yoga asana *can* and *should* be practiced by everybody— LITERALLY EVERY BODY. Once we recognize that the mainstream images of yoga are merely marketing, the same way they market lipstick and yogurt, then we can change the perception of what a "yogi" physically looks like.

Amen, Jessamyn!

It's easy and inexpensive to get started. I recommend that you start with a couple of beginner classes (there are studios everywhere; look online for one near you). You don't need any equipment—most studios have a mat you can borrow, or you can always ask a friend (because yes, ALL OF YOUR FRIENDS ARE DOING YOGA). Many studios allow you to pay for a class at a time, and most offer beginner's specials. There are many different kinds of yoga you can try, but hatha is generally good for someone who is new to the discipline. You don't have to wear or bring anything fancy, just comfortable clothes that aren't too baggy; you will want to be able to see the contours of your body when you look in the mirror to make sure you are doing poses correctly. Some people bring a little towel or a bottle of water, but beginner's yoga generally doesn't get you too sweaty. (And if you really can't get to a studio, try online classes from the comfort of your home. They're good for consistent practice, or when you're in a pinch. For example, when I recently suffered through a round of panic attacks while putting up a new Off-Broadway show, Adriene's routines at yogawithadriene.com and on YouTube totally saved me.)

A lot of people are nervous to try yoga because they think it's going to be religious, or that it will involve a lot of chanting in a language you've never heard before. Well, the poses have Sanskrit names, but most of them have English translations ("utkatasana" is chair pose, for example). You might be asked to make a noise that sounds like "Ohhhm," and yes, that's chanting, but it's really just a peaceful, centering thing that does not involve you converting to Hinduism. At the end of the class you may be asked to press your palms together and say "Namaste" (Nah-mah-stay), which pretty much means, "The divine within me recognizes the divine within you." It's just a mutual respect thing, and it sort of sets the tone. But the best thing about it (and yoga in general) is that if you feel uncomfortable, you don't have to do it.

The very best option, if you can afford it and if you're interested, is taking a private yoga lesson—even just one—with a teacher in your area. It's a really good way to make sure you are in alignment. You can even film it on your cell phone. That's what my mom did. She recorded the session, then took it home so she could remember the correct posture the next time she did those poses.

Once you've tried a few classes and understand some of the basic poses (PS: don't be freaked out if the teacher tries to give you some adjustments while you're doing the poses; there's no judgment, she's just helping you), you can try it on your own, following along with a book or a DVD, while you watch yourself in a mirror. (Tara Stiles's downloads are amazing: "Basics" and "Gentle" are a great place to start, or you can try her "Strong" one-hour power class if you really want your ass kicked. And "Relax" is wonderful for a little yoga hit at night before bed. Tara also has a great free video on YouTube for yoga that calms you pre-snooze.)

I have an awesome friend I work with named Jess, who runs a company called Yada Yada Yoga. She helps match up wannabe yoga students with quality yoga teachers. That's how I was lucky enough to meet a very cool yoga teacher, Jen, here in LA. I (not so) jokingly call Jen my "spirit animal." She's taught me a lot about yoga and breathing, and I love working with her. She's always very encouraging and empowering; she pushes me but never makes me feel like I have to do something challenging right away, like a handstand. She's big on moderation—and if she wants to have a burger and fries, that yogi's gonna eat them. Like the best yoga teachers, she brings a lot of love and intention to her practice, putting students in a good mental place before they even begin.

Here are some wise words from Jess and Jen (some of them are very complimentary to me—thanks guys, I'm honored!):

Yoga helps people live balanced lives. Flexibility of the body translates to flexibility in all things: relationships, life changes, schedules, travel, and even the way food affects you (and this is a short list, believe us). When we started doing yoga we didn't overthink it, we just kept showing up. Years later, we live with open hearts. The practice gives a focus on forgiveness and compassion toward ourselves and others, and immeasurable strength of mind and body. The flexibility teaches us that we simply cannot do every pose, and that is perfectly fine.

Most Yada Yada Yoga clients we meet with work very hard at what they do, and we believe yoga should not be another stress in life. It should be an approach to releasing tensions from work, while adding a healthy amount of challenge to make us stronger, and providing enough focus on breathing to take our minds beyond the physical.

When people ask us where to begin, we always say just sit down, close your eyes, and simply feel yourself breathing. Everybody has five minutes a day they could give themselves to connect the mind to the body and just feel the breath. Yes, this is the most basic suggestion, but so many people overwhelm themselves, and just getting started in this simple way is how you become flexible.

If you're looking to start a simple practice, consider the following series of poses. A good theory is to do each one for at least five breaths:

Sukhasana—Easy Seat (seated cross-legged; sit on folded blanket for more support), close your eyes and feel yourself breathe ten deep breaths
Balasana—Child's Pose
Bidalasana—Cat/Cow Pose
Adho Mukha Svanasana—Downward Facing Dog Pose
Prasarita Padottanasana—Wide Legged Forward Bend Pose
Viparita Karani—Legs Up the Wall Pose
Savasana—Corpse Pose

Each person truly is unique, so different types of yoga appeal to each of us. There is a vast amount of sequences, pose variations, adjustments, and preferences when it comes to yoga. That's why working with a teacher you trust is really beneficial.

We have watched Beth's poses transition from learning and trying, to graceful and flowing. Challenging poses do not come easily, but Beth uses her positive spirit to avoid beating herself up if she doesn't get it immediately, which is essential for change. We move on and keep going, and each day she decides to do the work that matters. This choice helps her find eloquent balance . . . and that is exactly what we love about yoga for ourselves.

Beth has the best attitude, and we believe that is exactly what has taken her so far in her practice. No matter how busy her schedule, Beth constantly shows up to her mat, to her breath, and to herself, and that kind of dedication always yields results. Keep showing up. It's the most important ingredient for everlasting growth and transformation.

Just as with Beth, each day will be different on your mat, and that is perfectly fine and healthy. Keep practicing with your best attitude. We become the measure of how we spend every day. A little does go a long way.

There are times when I try to shake off stress with exercise. For example, late one Friday afternoon, I got in a fight on the phone with my mom over our plans for Christmas. I was already so stressed out because it was the first Christmas that I was hosting at my own house, and I was annoyed that we had to rush around to make a certain Mass she wanted to attend. Admittedly, we were both tired after super-long weeks at work. We ended our call by snapping at each other and hanging up the phone. I was infuriated . . . but I went upstairs to my room and downloaded the hardest yoga class I could find. An hour later I not only called my mom to apologize but all of a sudden I felt so excited and happy about how special it was to host Christmas dinner. The combination of yoga, revelation, and peace with my mom melted the stress away.

OTHER BIG BREATH OPTIONS

As far as I'm concerned, you could do yoga every day and never get bored. But to keep things interesting, and to make sure you're moving your body in different delightful ways, here are some other Big Breath options that you can explore:

Walking/Power Walking/Running

Going for a nice stroll, a good, brisk walk, or a run is such a win-win. You don't need fancy equipment or a gym to just put on shoes and put one foot in front of the other. Cue up some music or an audiobook to keep you company if you need it, give yourself a few minutes to stretch, and just GO. Some of my friends who walk and run outside enjoy tracking their course on apps like MapMyWalk, or keep track of their exercise with a pedometer or a Fitbit. I love getting outside to work out, but if you are going to do your walking or running on a treadmill, you can mix it up a little bit by choosing one of the preset courses that give you some options to climb hills or do a little interval training.

Biking

Long-distance biking is a terrific workout, and it gives you a whole new way of looking at the world as it goes whizzing by. Just be sure to take the appropriate safety precautions, like wearing a helmet and reflectors. And please, don't be one of those people biking and talking on your phone at the same time (really? Life's too short). You can also grab your bike any old time to run errands or go visit a neighbor, instead of driving your car down the street. If you're on a stationary or recumbent bike at the gym, try some of the preprogrammed courses or offer to "race" the biker next to you.

Swimming

Give life to your inner mermaid and get in the pool. It's not always easy to swim if you're not in a warm climate, but you can look for community centers and gyms that feature indoor pools. Aside from being an amazing cardiovascular workout, there's something really peaceful and meditative about being in water and the cool silence under the surface. When you get the chance to take a dip in the ocean or a lake, go for it. It's a wonderful opportunity to connect with nature, and you might even forget that you're exercising.

WHEN IN DOUBT, DANCE IT OUT

When nothing's working for you . . . when you just can't imagine a way to get yourself up and at 'em . . . I have a surefire suggestion: dance.

Michael and I once went on vacation in Mexico, and we'll never forget this little girl we saw there. She couldn't have been more than four or five. There was a mariachi band playing at the hotel, and we would go watch her dance. She was SO into dancing by herself in front of the band, turning and jumping in her own little dance world. It was amazing and delightful, and such a pure thing to watch this young girl do that. I thought, "I wish I could live my life more like that . . . like I don't care."

Because we all start like that—twirling and dancing like no one's watching. Then one day, we start to become self-conscious, wondering, *Is my boob hanging out?* Or, *Am I off rhythm?* (Okay, if your boob is hanging out, just pop it back in there.)

So I tell you: Dance alone in your room in your PJs. Nothing feels better. If you are feeling bad, turn on your favorite music and spin like crazy. It will elevate your mood, and guess what: That's cardio, baby!

Songs That Make Me Feel . . .

Music is a really big motivator for me—not just when it comes to exercise but for just about anything throughout the day. I play music while I'm working out, cooking, and driving in my car. Sometimes when I'm stressing out, all I need to do is pop in a pair of headphones (or better yet, crank up the speakers) and listen to a favorite tune to recalibrate my whole system. Whether it's a moment of great doubt—or total celebration—I find that music gets me right on track. Here are some of my favorites when I feel . . .

HAPPY!
> Dolly Parton, "9 to 5"

DANCE-Y!
> Montell Jordan, "This Is How We Do It"

SAD, BUT GOOD SAD
> Lady Antebellum, "Need You Now"

SAD, BUT BAD SAD
> Emmylou Harris, "Orphan Girl"

BROADWAY-READY
> *Thoroughly Modern Millie* soundtrack (both the movie version with Julie Andrews and the Broadway revival soundtrack with the incredible Sutton Foster)

EMPOWERED
> Anything Beyoncé!

LONELY AND NEEDIN' SOME LOVIN'
> Mumford & Sons' *Babel* album (always, without fail, any time of day or night)

ENERGIZED
> Jay Z featuring Justin Timberlake, "Holy Grail" (or any old-school Jay Z, even with the hyphen)

SENTIMENTAL
Bon Jovi, "Livin' on a Prayer" (my dad and I used to belt it out on road trips)
CALM & PEACEFUL
Swell Season, Hozier, or Sam Smith
KARAOKE-WINNING
My go-to with a boy is always "Summer Nights" from *Grease*—I've karaoke'd it with Jonathan Kite (a.k.a. Oleg from my show), Darren Criss from *Glee*, and Max Greenfield from *New Girl*. My gal karaoke pick is "Alone" by Heart. I've even Mariah Karaoke'd that song with Oscar-winner Amy Adams! She has an insanely amazing voice and killed the high harmony.
LIKE, MUST SING ALOUD
Anything from Taylor Swift's *1989*
UNBEATABLE
Survivor, "Eye of the Tiger" from *Rocky*—of course!

WHAT TO DO WHEN . . .

By this point you're realizing that exercise isn't just something you want to do . . . it's something you *have* to do. You may actually find that after you miss a day or two of your moves, your body and mind really feel it. I know I feel more sluggish and stiff, and kind of overall out of it, when I can't make time to move. But even with the best intentions, life gets in the way. So here are a few suggestions for when you're stuck but you still want to get a move on.

Here's what to do when you're . . .

. . . stuck at the airport.

Instead of sitting at your gate, move. Pretend you're a mall walker and really go for it. You may be carrying some heavy stuff, but use it as weights and get your blood pumping. At the very least, take the long way to the gate instead of using the moving sidewalks. Also keep in mind that over 200 airports in the US and Canada now have workout rooms and yoga studios (check airportgyms.com for a full list).

If you're at the airport in Seoul, you can ice skate (!), and if you're in Munich, be sure to play mini-golf with the kids.

. . . on an airplane.

You definitely have to stretch your legs on an airplane, even if it's just walking up and down the aisle. Larger planes have galleys where you can really stretch out with some basic bends and twists. In your seat, you can do small movements like putting your fist between your knees, squeezing your legs together, and releasing. And if ever there was a time to Kegel . . .

. . . at a hotel.

Most hotels have gym facilities; just call to investigate in advance. I'd also recommend bringing your resistance bands or TRX from your home gym (see page 190) and keeping up your routine. That will give you lots of options and take up almost no room in your suitcase.

. . . without gym shoes.

Oh no! You're traveling and you forgot your sneakers! No prob. You can do one of your living room workouts, no shoes required—including a bunch of burpees and squats (the same goes for if you show up at the gym sans shoes). You could also do some of the yoga poses included on page 216. If you're near a beach, try running or walking in the surf for a real challenge.

. . . on vacation.

You're on vacay—of course you don't want a task; you want to relax. So switch gears and do some stretching and breathing, do some yoga poses (see page 216), or try some of the meditation exercises you'll find in the next section.

. . . at a Bar Mitzvah.

Hora, baby!

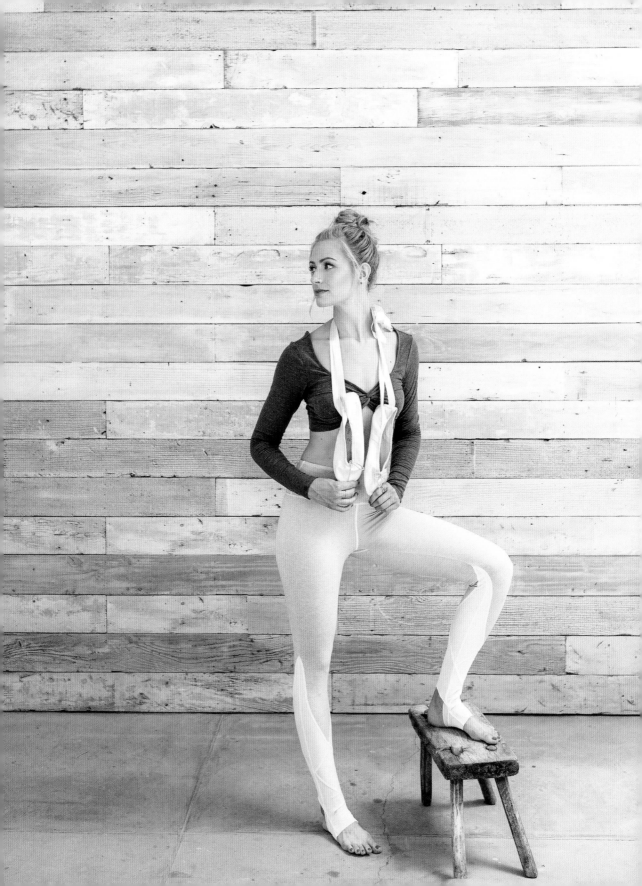

CHAPTER 11

GROUP MOVES

I know how hard it is to amp up your level of exercise—but I swear, once I really got it into my system, I really wanted to do it. I also found that it helped if I was having fun—I would forget it was fitness and just start enjoying myself. For most people, that starts with getting friends involved. So, for example, if you've got a regular book club, you may want to mix it up and work out together before you break down that month's read. If you're looking to meet new people, check out local leagues and meet-up groups. Here are some ways to turn fitness from something on your checklist into a social event.

TENNIS, ANYONE?

I recently fell in love with tennis. Not only does it feel incredible to be doing something competitively (and I am competitive; let's just say that when my little sister beat me once in Wii Tennis on Nintendo, I *might* have thrown and broken things), but it's also an amazing workout without being an ACTUAL workout. It's social and fun. You can play with friends, family, or sig Os and laugh . . . while fixing the dimples in your butt. Seriously. I see better results after playing tennis three times a week than I do lifting weights. It's cardio, booty, and core all in one.

You can learn some crazy life lessons from tennis as well. You have to stay calm and in the moment while under pressure (for someone with severe panic attacks, this is a great lesson). I play much better when I'm calm and letting go; I also do my best professional work when I apply the same philosophy. Also, after a long freakin' day, nothing feels better than whacking that little bundle of yellow fuzz. What a release. Not to mention the FASHION. Tennis whites? Hello!!! So chic. I feel like Chad and Barbie, going to have a game of doubles and a martini at the country club, even when I'm just going to play at a public court at Griffith Park with a can of LaCroix.

Speaking of the snoot factor: Tennis traditionally has a "fancy pants," must-have-money-to-play kind of vibe. So not true. There are public courts in pretty much every city (check your city's recreation website). Serena and Venus Williams's father taught them to play from reading a book. After you screen a little YouTube and flip through a couple of books, you can go to the public court and work on your serve and stroke.

HAVE SOME CLASS

Do a little research and look into classes in your neighborhood that you and your pals might enjoy doing together. Zumba? Dance? Spin? Personally I'm in love with a class here in LA called Ballet Bodies, taught by Andie Hecker, where we do ballet moves and Pilates. When I go with friends, we have so much fun that we forget we are even exercising in the first place. It also takes me back to childhood dance class. Oh, to feel young again!

CROSSFIT/BOOT CAMP/SPINNING

If you're looking for action where you can soak up the energy of a group while working at your own challenging pace, try CrossFit, boot camp, or spinning classes. My friend Matt, who I mentioned earlier, has gotten me into the boot camp scene lately (he's a trainer at Barry's Bootcamp in NYC). I dig this kind of workout because I never, ever get bored. The hour-long session zips by so quickly that by the time I'm over sprinting or hating the crunches, I'm on to the next move. I love that the lighting is dark so no one can see how high up your treadmill is, or if you sweat through your white top (and you will SWEAT!). Also, the music is always fantastic, and the trainers get you pumped! Workouts are made up of a half hour of interval cardiovascular routines on the treadmill, followed by a half hour of strength training with free weights, resistance bands, medicine balls, and other equipment. They mix up the segments and trainers so that no class during the week is ever the same.

GROUP STAND-UP PADDLING

For about $10 you can rent a board and go for it. I like it because it's the equivalent of riding a bike on the water—everyone can do it once you get the hang of it. Not only is it an incredible workout for your legs and core, but you can also chat while you do it, like going on a hike. And if you get tired, just lie down for a sec in the sunshine . . . dreamy.

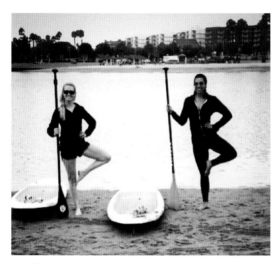

Paddling with my college roommate Courtney. Well, it's pre-paddle.

TAKE A HIKE

Seriously, what's better than getting out into the great outdoors? Bringing some friends along and making it a social event! I just did a five-day hiking trip through Point Reyes in Northern California with my closest friends. We hiked fifteen miles a day with twenty-five-pound packs on our backs. It was *Wild*, and wild. Our guide told us to keep our packs light—no cosmetics or toiletries. Of course, I threw in some tinted moisturizer, deodorant, and three face wipes—no regrets. Oh, and hand sanitizer. You're peeing in the woods, come on! But I really appreciated my community of friends, the beauty of nature, and the ability to step away from media—social and otherwise—for just a few days.

Of course, you don't have to make an overnight event out of it . . . grab a friend and take a quick hike near your home if you have some interesting terrain nearby. And if your terrain is not that stimulating—no wide-open spaces, hills, or forests to explore—you can make even a walk around the neighborhood more interesting if you bring a pal along.

A LEAGUE OF YOUR OWN

Join a local league! Kickball, basketball, softball . . . foosball, if you insist. That's what I did when I first got out of school and had no money for the gym or for classes. In addition to keeping you in shape and giving you a workout, a league provides an opportunity to meet new people and bond over your love of the game. Not to mention the bar crawl after a championship win . . .

EVEN MORE MOTIVATION

Once your workout is super social, you'll start to forget the real reason you started to group train in the first place . . . was it for the fitness, or for the fun? Either way you're reaping huge benefits. And whenever your motivation starts to flag, call on one of your workout buddies to help you get it going again. Their company or their wise words could make a difference when you need it most.

I was on a run with my friend Jessy once when she started talking to herself (and I guess to me). She was ordering, "Harder! Stronger! Faster!" and "Make it happen, make it happen!" At first she was cracking me up . . . then I realized, she was helping us run farther and harder. I couldn't believe it! When we were done with the run I said, "J, I think most people would consider that a little cray . . . where did your inner drill sergeant come from?" She responded, "I read this study that said that athletes who practiced encouraging self-talk, and did things like thinking positively about themselves and the task they had to do, went harder for much longer . . . which not only makes you a badass by increasing endurance, but it also makes doing your sweaty thing seem less difficult." She gave me something essential I needed to make my run better. Best of all, it was free! Thanks, Jessy!

Here are a few other ideas to help you and your peeps keep up your heart rates with workouts:

Vision Board Parties

If you are about to embark on a new workout endeavor, gather some girlies to-gether first to make a vision board, or a collection of inspiring pictures, quotes, you name it to help keep you on track with your goals. Get a bunch of magazines, poster board, tape, and glue, and dig around for things that speak to you. Write

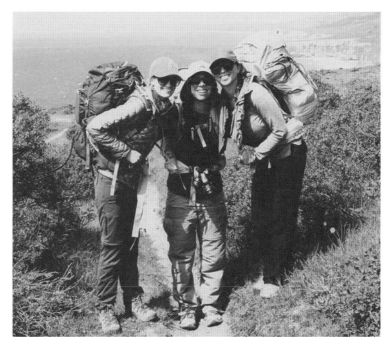

Fresh air, friends, being the one who's in focus—what could be better?

A SHOUT-OUT TO GETTING OUTSIDE

I'm a big fan of exercising outdoors. It's not just fun—it may actually be better for you than a trip to the gym. Here's why:

- Research indicates that outdoor exercise not only boosts energy and vitality but also decreases anger, depression, and tension.
- If you feel self-conscious exercising around others, the great outdoors does not give a rat's ass about what you look like or how well you do your moves.
- Studies show that people generally enjoy exercising outside more than inside, and when you are having a good time you are more likely to do it again.
- Exercising in the sunshine (with appropriate sunscreen) gives you a burst of vitamin D3, which supports bone health and metabolic function. Exposure to the sun during the day is also supposed to help you sleep better at night.
- Best of all: Working out in nature is FREE.

down your goals next to those items and paste them on the board. I did this with my friend Marley, who is a stuntwoman. We found pictures of strong women to post on our boards as a daily reminder that we kick butt.

Money Jar Jam

When I was training for a half marathon, I sometimes had a really, really tough time dragging myself out of bed in the morning for my run. My creative friend Courtney gave me a great idea. She said, "Beth, I want you to decorate a mason jar with fitspiration photos, then after finishing your run, put a couple of bucks in it. Once the jar is full, you can treat yourself to a new adorable workout top or shorts, or a delicious fancy cheat-day meal at your favorite restaurant." Will do, Court! Another cool idea? Save the dough and put all the money from training toward a vacation you may not have been fit enough to attempt before, like hiking Yosemite, taking a cycling tour of Oregon, swimming in a coral reef in Hawaii . . . man, I really want to do that!

This Used to Be My Playground

If the workouts start feeling like a drag, get a group of grown-ups together and let your inner children out! Play. Just like you did when you were little. Hide-and-seek, scavenger hunts, tag, homemade obstacle courses, Frisbee, tug o' war . . . maybe stay away from dodgeball—wasn't much fun then, still won't be now. Take a minute when the games are over to stand as a group and remind yourselves of the importance of play. Be grateful to be in bodies that are able to jump, run, and slide. Then get back to business, knowing that fun is always part of the process.

AND THEN . . . LIFE HAPPENS: DEALING WITH AN INJURY

You're on a roll, you're moving, and you finally see what all the fuss is about with this whole exercise thing. You feel stronger, more energetic, and more confident. But then it happens—you get injured. Believe me, I've been there. I recently had a hip injury. It started as a terrible stabbing pain I felt in my groin every time my left foot hit the ground, and it totally waylaid me. I was enormously disappointed because I had spent two months training for a marathon. I'd set a goal and I'd stuck to it. I was getting used to waking up early, and my body was starting to crave that runner's high. When the doctor told me I couldn't work out for two weeks, my body got depressed. It missed moving. I missed it, too. It sucked. Luckily, I met a great physical therapist who helped me gain the strength I needed through weight training and Pilates. He also eventually cleared me to do boxing, which gave me the same high as running. He told me that my injury was a long time coming and was most likely due to the way my growth plate formed from the high-impact soccer I had played as a kid. He said the fact that I lasted until thirty was amazing; my body was simply not built for distance running.

I had to face the facts: My dream of running a marathon was not going to happen. I let myself feel bad for a minute and then . . . okay, fine. I had to find new goals, create new ways of competing with myself and others. Whatever I do, I'm not giving up. *American Ninja Warrior*, here I come. Or something like that.

If you're laid low by an injury, don't let it get you down. Put in the work you need to get healthy, and then reevaluate if the exercise you're doing is truly good for your body. I recommend working with an expert, like a physical therapist, who can help you understand your body's natural strengths and weaknesses. But whatever you do, don't give up! You're going to get back in the game.

THE TOTAL PACKAGE

You see, there are tons of ways of working out that don't require inducing a heart attack or even going to a gym. It's all about balance. It's okay to say, "Today I'm just going to do my Meh, then watch some TV and break out the medicine ball or workout bands." I guarantee, you will feel better than when you started. Fine, so you may not reach your specific goal tomorrow, but you will FEEL BETTER, and that's the whole point—to improve your quality of life.

And should life happen—you get busy, you get sick, you get injured, you have to travel—then you just start over again. Small steps, bigger breaths, invite others. Instead of feeling like an order, it's going to feel like a relief, and eventually— sooner than you think—like a happy, healthy way of life.

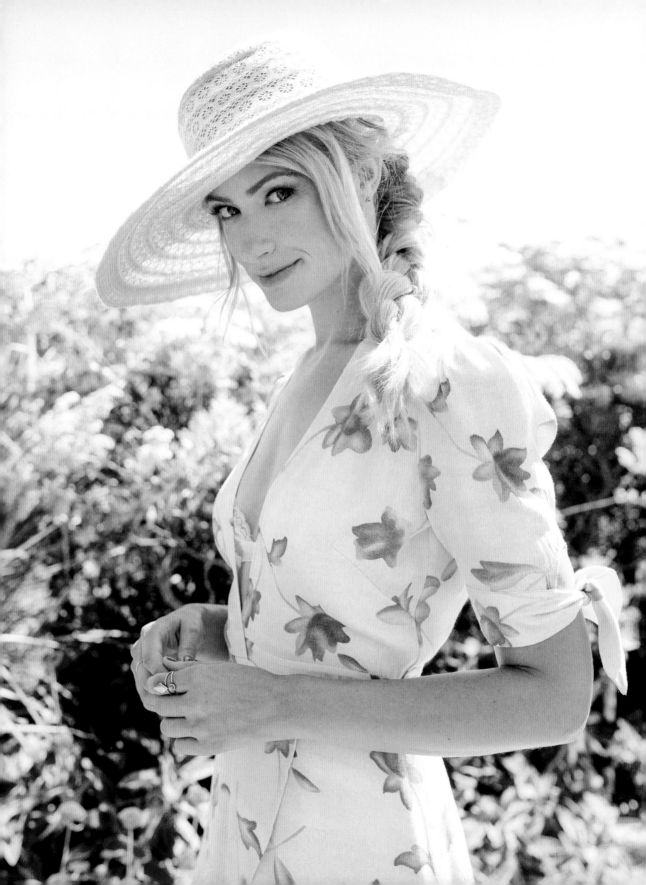

Part III

LOVE YOUR LIFE

EVOLVING FROM MANIC PANIC TO CHILL CHICK

As a kid, I had a lot of anxiety. And I was a total hypochondriac. I was this little peanut, worrying that I had something wrong with my heart or that I was dying of cancer. Sometimes I'd lose my breath to the point that I was almost hyperventilating. I had a terrible bout of this behavior after my sophomore year of college, and my little sister, Emily (who legitimately had asthma), asked me, "What are you thinking about?" I didn't think I was thinking about anything . . . but Emily was always intuitive that way. She calmly and rationally explained, "You're just having a panic attack."

Panic attacks are no joke, of course. And whether or not you have a good "reason" for going into full-on panic mode, your body responds with a surge of adrenaline so high that some people think they are having a heart attack. Your heart races. It feels like you can't breathe. You may become disoriented or confused. While I always tended toward anxiety, my panic attacks increased exponentially in college. It took me a while to figure out what escalated things, but a lot of soul searching led me back to a flight I was on that had to do an emergency landing. In that moment, thinking the plane was going to crash, I realized I had no control. For some people that's comforting. For me, it set off a response mechanism in my system that downward spiraled until I was a lost cause. For a full year, I wouldn't fly. And while I eventually got back on a plane, it took me years to find a real way to combat my anxiety.

There are all different ways to deal with panic, stress, anxiety, and fear. Medication and therapy are common solutions. But I found something that doesn't involve putting chemicals in my body or shelling out major bucks for counseling. It was meditation that helped curb my panic attacks and gave me a true sense of well-being. That's why it is the third element in my three-part get-your-shit-together plan (after changing the way you eat and exercising).

Whether you are crippled by feelings of anxiety or you are just looking to gently shift your outlook to one of positivity and good health, some practice of mindfulness or meditation will help you. It doesn't even really need to be full-on meditation that you do, but some element of activity that's mindful, focused on thoughts and feelings. The best part is that there's no right or wrong way to engage in mindfulness. "Morning pages" are awesome—that's when you wake up and free-write a few pages on any subject you want, without editing yourself as you go (see page 238). Journaling in general is a genius way to keep track of what you've done and assess yourself in a new light. Some people find inner peace through prayer. I grew up Catholic—remember my great aunt Meme, the nun? While the practice of Mass didn't really resonate with me, I loved the music and felt like it gave me a higher connection and a real buzz. I have that same feeling when I finish a meditation session.

Before you even dip your toe into the mindful zone, prepare your body and mind to make the shift to welcoming peace and positivity into your life. Here are a few things you can try . . .

TEN TEENSY-TINY THINGS YOU CAN DO TO MAKE YOUR DAY BETTER

1. Start your day drinking water with lemon. It cleanses toxins from your system, gives you a boost of vitamin C and potassium, and refreshes your body. BONUS: Drink your lemon water outside while watching the sunrise for an even more invigorating start to a crazy day. On filming days I make it a point to begin my morning outside. Breathing in the fresh air helps me feel centered and happy and ready to take on the day ahead. Which leads me to . . .

2. Work out outside. Take your weights to your front lawn, go for a brisk walk, ride a skateboard . . . just do something outside. Sweat for twenty minutes in the great outdoors. You'll feel more relaxed and more at peace, and you'll get a burst of immune system–boosting vitamin D.

3. Commit to one leafy green. Whether it's in a smoothie, a juice, a salad at lunch . . . just eat at least one a day. That's how I started craving greens. I noticed I felt better just hours after I ate them, so I wanted to down them more and more. Those feel-goods aren't just in your mind—chlorophyll is a natural mood booster.

4. Cook dinner at home. Do it with a significant other, friends, or solo . . . but leave your cell phones locked away in another room. Drink wine, play music, dance around the kitchen, and talk to each other without checking your Instafeed.

5. Take five minutes of quiet time. Sit in a dimly lit room, in silence, for at least five minutes. Taking just five minutes to calm your mind and body will make a huge difference in your outlook, your energy, and your general feeling of wellness. (Now that I do twenty minutes twice a day of transcendental meditation, my body craves it like it's a steaming-hot pizza—more on that later.)

6. Be kind. Smile at a stranger on the subway, donate a dollar to an organization that approaches you on the street, or ask the grocery checkout gal how her week is going. Just be kind.

7. Get creative. Remember how often we drew pictures, sang a song with Mom, or wrote in a diary when we were kids? Bring that back. Write in a journal, buy an adult coloring book and go to town, pick up an instrument, create your own recipe, or build some DIY furniture—just get those creative juices flowing. It's not just for kicks; research shows that being creative makes you feel happier, less anxious, and more resilient. You can lean on creativity to help you solve problems in unusual ways. That lowers stress, leading to a healthier body and mind. For even more tips on how to incorporate creativity into your day, check out page 238.

8. Take a bath. Light a candle and add some salts, essential oils, or bubbles, and it will feel like you're on vacation in your own home. BONUS: Bathing before bed will help you get a more restful night's sleep.

9. Take a risk/commit to a challenge. Boost your confidence by speaking up in a meeting you wouldn't normally feel comfortable contributing to, asking your boss for that raise you deserve, or making a plan to conquer your fear of heights. I'm getting my confidence on right now by taking rock-climbing lessons—it's thrilling and challenging and scary and wonderful!

10. Take a moment. Before bed, think of all the things you were grateful for that day. It will definitely make for a better night's sleep.

HERE'S HOW YOU START: BIT BY BIT

Eventually, you'll be able to get to this place, this calm, Zen place, in the center of the mania that is your life. And just like eating . . . just like exercising . . . the best way to make changes that will last for a lifetime is to start with just a little something.

DAY ONE: When you have a moment by yourself—preferably right when you wake up—sit up and place your feet on the floor and your hands in your lap. Take a deep breath and hold it in for ten seconds. Now slowly let it out. See if you can feel the way your lungs filled and emptied, or the way your shoulders came down from that tight spot in your neck. Carry on with your morning.

DAY TWO: Set your alarm for five minutes earlier than usual. Do the same breathing exercise you did on Day One. After you let that breath out and notice any changes in your body, sit for two more minutes and think about your intentions for the day.

DAY THREE: Same as Day Two. Add an extra breath before you go to bed at night.

DAY FOUR: **Same as Day Three.**

DAY FIVE: **Same as Days Three and Four, but add this exercise:** Take ten minutes to write down a list of things you are grateful for. They can be big or small. Keep this list with you.

DAY SIX: **Repeat your breathing exercises and intention setting. Today's exercise is to send positive vibes to someone else.** Give someone a compliment, think about someone who needs good energy, or silently send some well wishes to that tired-looking person sitting across from you on the bus. Either way, send the good stuff out.

DAY SEVEN: **Same breathing and intention work, but your exercise today is to direct those good vibes inward.** Think kindly about yourself. Make a list of three good things about you, and give yourself some love for those things.

DAY EIGHT: **Instead of one big morning breath, breathe calmly in and out for two minutes.** (You can set an alarm if you want to keep your eyes closed, or avoid looking at a clock.) Make sure at one point in the day you send good vibes to someone else as well as give some lovin' to yourself.

DAY NINE: **In addition to your morning breath, intention setting, and good vibes, set aside ten to twenty minutes today for a guided meditation** (you can find a list of these on page 253).

DAY TEN: **During your morning breath, think about the last nine days.** Do you notice a difference in the way you feel, in your behavior? Are you a little slower to beep your horn in traffic? Are you a little more patient when you can afford to be? Are you a little more generous to yourself when you make a mistake? If you can answer "yes" to any of these questions or others like them, then you are on your way to becoming a more mindful, me-toxed human being.

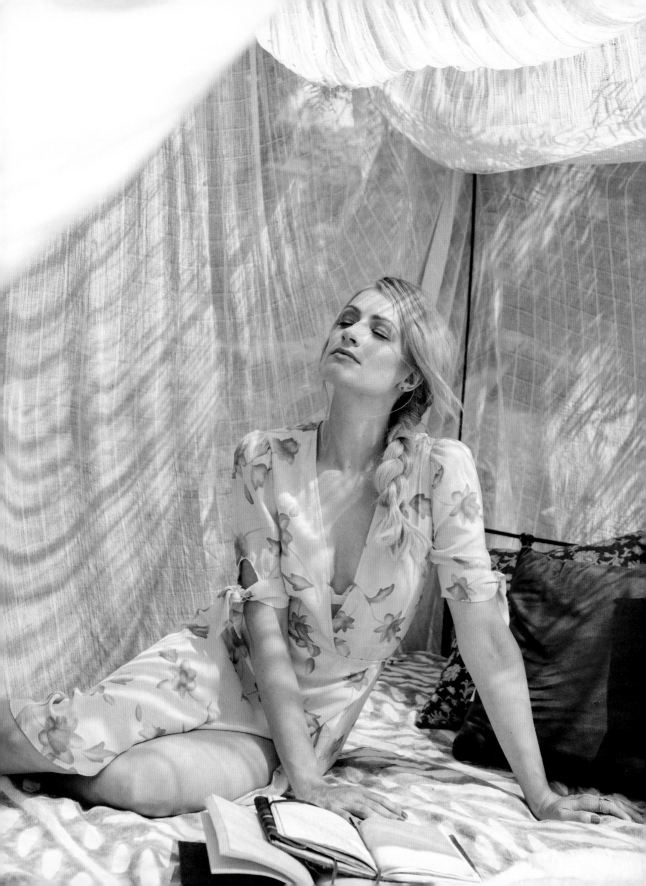

CHAPTER 12

BEING MINDFUL

What is "mindfulness," anyway? It's a word (and frankly, kind of an annoying word) that gets tossed around a lot. Jon Kabat-Zinn is a biologist who first coined the term *mindfulness* in the '70s, and he defined it as a state of mind in which you're actually paying attention on purpose and being present without passing judgment. It seems like a trendy thing, but it really comes from centuries-old Buddhist styles of meditation. To me, being mindful is just being more conscious or aware of something. And once you're aware of something—a problem, a need, a change that has to be made—it gets a little harder to ignore. That can be something as small as, "I'm on my last roll of toilet paper" to, "THE PLANET IS MELTING!" (Note: One of these problems is easier to fix than the other.)

The researched benefits of mindfulness are ridiculous: It improves attention, reduces stress, regulates emotion, increases levels of compassion and empathy, can improve sensory processing, and may relieve some side effects of aging (like memory loss). Mindfulness techniques can be used to treat aggression, ADHD, and anxiety. So looking at that list . . . why wouldn't you want to be mindful?

There are lots of easy ways to invite mindfulness into your daily life. For example, every time you look in the mirror, fight your instinct to be critical and give yourself a compliment instead. Every time you wash your hands, notice them and the way they move and work. Take a sec to feel gratitude for having hands that can do so much cool stuff. Every time you turn on your car, send a happy thought to someone you care about. Sounds cheesy, but in the same way you can try to hex someone with a nasty glance, you might as well turn that frown upside down. Or every time you hear the word "Kardashian," take a deep breath. Because we all need to.

I've tried lots of different tools to bring more mindfulness, creativity, and peace into my life. If you'd like to upgrade from happy thoughts and deep breaths to an actual mindfulness practice, here are some of my favorite methods:

Creativity

Getting in touch with your creative self is a wonderful way to bring consciousness and awareness into your life . . . and you won't even realize you're doing it. Experiencing art is a great way to start—but sitting in a movie theater or watching a TV show isn't ideal if that's something you do all the time. Take yourself on a date to a museum. Go see live theater. Or put headphones on and listen to music that's usually not on your playlist—classical if you're a rap fan, rap if you dig classical.

You can also engage in art yourself. Draw or paint, freestyle or in a coloring book (there's a reason those adult coloring books are a big hit). Start a DIY home décor project or try knitting (I get lost in the repetitive clicking of the needles, and I love it). If you're a parent, sit down with your kid the next time she's drawing or stamping and make her a picture for once. Sing a song in the shower when no one's listening. Learn the instrument you always meant to take up (piccolo, here I come!). If you have some friends who play, ask them if you can join in on a casual sesh, even if you're just drumming in your lap or dinging the triangle.

I also highly recommend a strategy that many of my friends learned from a book called *The Artist's Way: A Spiritual Path to Higher Creativity*. The book's author, Julia Cameron, suggests you start your day by writing "morning pages." Basically, you just sit down and start writing until three pages are filled up. It doesn't have to be anything brilliant, and you don't have to have any particular goal in mind. Writing for writing's sake opens your mind and unconsciously takes you places you want to go. So get yourself a little journal and, at the top of your day, scribble away.

Journaling

Here's another use for that journal: journaling. Every day, write something in your journal. You can just jot down a couple of things that happened to you that day.

It's super fun to go back later and say, "Wow, did I really walk up to Justin Timberlake and say, 'Oh my God, you're Justin Timberlake'?" (Yes, I did.) You can also use your journal to make lists, write down pros and cons for decision making, collect quotes or snippets of dialogue you like, keep track of ideas . . . and you may find that that little collection of notes turns into a legit creative outlet for you.

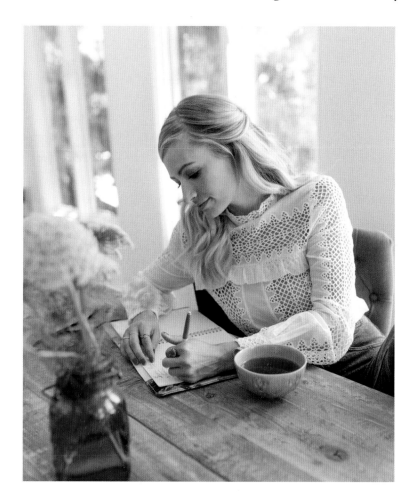

Visualization

Pro athletes I admire channel this brand of positivity and the law of attraction. US Women's Soccer champ Carli Lloyd says before a game she visualizes herself scoring four or five goals and breaking records. She imagines the good and makes it happen. Not, "What if I trip?" or "Uh-oh, what if I get hurt?" But, "How many different ways can I own this game?" We can bring that same power to our lives. I visualize making a room full of people laugh before I tape a show. Or I picture myself nailing an audition. You can do this, too: Before you walk into that job interview, imagine yourself being offered the gig. Take the nervous energy you feel before a date and channel it into visualizing the great time you're going to have that night. It might not guarantee the outcome you want, but it will help set you up with confidence and positivity, which are very powerful forces.

Equine/Animal Therapy

Another sort of "meditation"—and an extremely helpful tool for my anxiety disorder—came from a very unexpected place when I began taking an equine-coaching/natural-horsemanship program at a ranch not far from my home. I've always loved horses, which were all over rural Virginia where I grew up. But I never rode because we couldn't afford it. When I booked *2 Broke Girls*, I discovered that

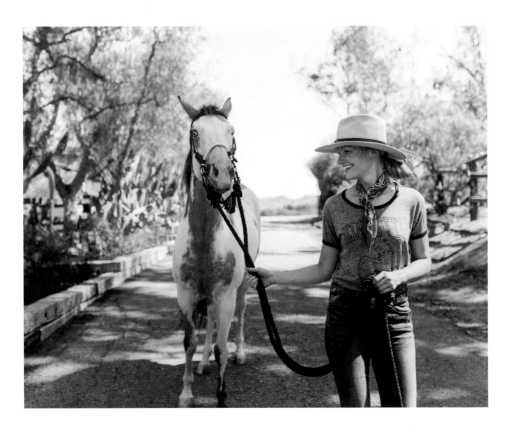

my other co-star besides Kat was a horse named Chestnut (long story). Kat and I absolutely fell in love with him. Having him on set brought instant joy and calm to both of us, and I wanted more of that in my life.

A few of my friends in California had tried and loved this all-natural equine-coaching program, so I signed up. The idea is that you're working with a horse "naturally," or without any tack, bit, or force, so the horse is only responding to you, in your full, most authentic, grounded human glory. The program explains itself this way: "[Horses] communicate best with our innate-self as they are herd animals, so their well-being depends on making sure the person they are following is genuine. Horses reflect non-judgmental feedback of what is clear and congruent in our presence and leadership and guide us to acknowledge what is ineffective in our personal actions and interactions. Once realized, we can see how trusting ourselves and being confident and true has a greater effect than how we usually operate." Sounds pretty great, right? It's said that you "pick a horse" based on what you need. I picked Bandit. Cassandra, the trainer, told me he was fearful and anxiety-ridden (sounds familiar), a little clumsy (figures), but very loyal and kind. A perfect fit for me.

Before beginning my session with Bandit, I learned that I had to let go of everything (the traffic on the way over, that fight with my boyfriend, my stress about work, etc.), or Bandit would get too nervous. I had to breathe deeply and ground myself in order to be most effective with the horse. If he got pushy or scared me in any way, my instinct was to get tense and anxious and start to freak out, which only exacerbated his forward energy. Forcing myself to slow down and relax, I was able to let go of tension and stand tall, feeling strong and connected to my surroundings. I've applied this kind of meditative, calm "energy" working with horses to other moments in my day-to-day life—especially the ones filled with fear, panic, and stress. In fact, I fell so in love with the program that I decided to rescue a horse of my own so that I could spend any and every day at the barn. Working with the ASPCA, I found her at a beautiful horse rescue in San Diego called Blue Apple Ranch. Her name is Belle. She's a six-year-old paint mare with blue eyes. I stare into them all the time, thinking to myself, "I came to help her . . . but she's helping me."

If you're not a horse person or don't have equine resources near you, consider volunteering at any kind of animal rescue program (a quick Internet search will get you going). There are shelters for household pets like dogs and cats, and farm-animal rescues are popping up all over the country, if you want to get your Old MacDonald on. You could also start with something simple like helping a busy or elderly neighbor out with their pet. Doing a good deed can lower stress and fill your soul, and you'll get some good animal nuzzling in at the same time.

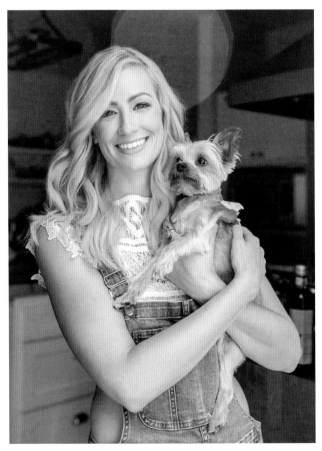

Betty!

Cooking

Don't forget that cooking is a kind of meditation! You sort of let yourself fall into the repetition of cleaning and chopping and following directions, and before you know it, your brain has made some interesting observations. That's why I recommend turning off your phone or your TV while you cook, so you can focus on the task at hand while also letting some interesting vibes settle in your brain. Be sure to use all five senses when you're cooking. Go through them one by one and notice the beautiful color of a bell pepper, the smell of garlic as it cooks, the taste of a chocolate chip. And let that extend into the act of eating your food and appreciating it in every way.

Engaging in Positivity

I believe in the power of positivity. The legendary actress Valerie Harper appeared on our show, and she taught me a lot about how to live life. Though she'd been diagnosed with brain cancer, her mind was strong and beautiful. She told me that every day she visualized her sickness being gone. And she has defied the odds . . . appearing on our show, on *Dancing with the Stars*, still making friends and giving great performances, making 'em laugh and making 'em cry. No matter what happens to Valerie, she is living an incredible life.

Now, when bad shit happens to me, I try to look at the upside. For example, the hip injury that I described on page 228. I was bummed about that. SO BUMMED. But I decided to see it as my body's . . . or a supreme being's . . . or the universe's way of telling me to slow down. Everyone told me that I was pushing myself too hard, but I wasn't ready to stop. No way was competitive Beth going to take a break! So my hip literally took a break for me. (I could look at the skin virus the same way. I was actively damaging myself, and my body said, "No way, Jose. You have to change your ways or you're going to regret it." And my body, in its infinite wisdom, was right.)

When you're faced with a challenge like a job interview, a big meeting with the boss, or giving a speech and find yourself in the zone of, "What if I suck? What if it's terrible?" pull out your positive power. Don't let your brain go to the negative place. It's all just your imagination anyway, so imagine yourself killing it! That's what I do with every audition. Before I walk into any party. Before I try something physical and new, like rollerblading. Make a little movie in your head, make it successful (and wear something fierce!), and let that positive vision guide you during the real thing.

Feeling Grateful

If there's one guiding element that's gotten me through some challenging times, it's gratitude. Gratitude isn't just a foo-foo thing—feeling grateful has been scientifically proven to improve health and overall well-being. Studies show that engaging in acts of gratitude, whether it's keeping a gratitude diary or writing a thank-you note, can make you feel better and even help lower levels of depression long after you've done them. It's true: A little bit of active gratitude can almost rewire your brain to feel extra thankful. Luckily, it's easy to cultivate gratitude and find ways to express it. Consider adding extra thank-yous to your day, whether it's at Starbucks or at the end of an e-mail. Send someone you care about a handwritten note thanking them for the influence they've had on your life—for no reason at all. Or keep an active and evolving gratitude list. Here's mine:

I'm grateful for . . .

My job. Not only does it put that roof over my head, but every day I get to do what I love to do, and that's a gift.

My family and my fiancé.

Having normal, sane, smart people around me. A lot of people in my business don't.

My house, which makes me feel proud and cozy and protected.

The zit on my face being significantly smaller than it was this morning.

Not having a nip slip in my menswear-inspired blazer on the red carpet last night.

Those twenty minutes I found to start a new book on my porch this evening.

My lentil burgers not falling apart when I made them.

Finding that parking spot (this is a major struggle in LA).

My dog Betty's unconditional love. I'm also grateful that she pooped (it matters more than you think).

The opportunity to share what I've learned with YOU.

CHAPTER 13

MEDITATION

As I continued to explore all different ways of bringing mindfulness into my life, I discovered another technique that has LITERALLY CHANGED EVERYTHING. More than the Vitamix. More than a thousand burpees. It's the key to a total me-tox: meditation. It's not just something I dig; it's something I need. Meditation has been proven to lower stress and improve physiological and mental health. If you're like me, you would probably want to know how this practice does all these amazing things. So I poked around a little bit and found some background on meditation from guru Deepak Chopra. His explanation is that meditation slows down your mind. And because your mind and your body are connected, your body also slows down, on a cellular level, giving it a chance to heal and regulate itself. (Scientists call this homeostatis. Is this all coming back to you from seventh-grade biology?)

Meditation can also lower the level of inflammation in the body. And because inflammation is a factor in almost every chronic illness, from autoimmune issues to arthritis, less inflammation is a really good thing. In addition to improving cardiovascular health and making you feel happier and more secure, meditation also lowers stress by amping up brain chemicals that give you the feel-goods, activates processes related to antiaging, and slows down processes that contribute to diseases like diabetes and Alzheimer's. Come on! You'd take it if it came in pill form—this just comes in chill form.

There are a zillion different ways to meditate, and I'm going to help you find the right one for you.

Beth, clearly this is the right step to take after improving the way I eat and the way I exercise.

It certainly is.

But . . .

Don't even go there. You're really going to give me the "but"?

I know it's going to be so good for me. But . . .

I CAN'T MEDITATE 'CAUSE . . .

I don't have time.

A little goes such a long way—even a minute will make a difference. You're going to schedule it in just like the other things you do for yourself. (As Deepak says, the people who say they don't have time for meditation are the people who need it most.)

I have a headache.

This could actually ease your headache. Or else, have a glass of water and maybe an Advil and let's get to it.

It's weird/goofy.

It's weird to you . . . but not to millions of people who do this every single day.

People are going to laugh at me.

First of all, you can do this privately and no one has to know. Second, haven't we learned by now that we don't care what other people think?

I can't sit still/I'm a go-go-go person.

Even the most energized people will benefit from a few moments of focus and stillness.

I don't know how.

I will show you!

There are too many noises and distractions.

You don't need privacy, darkness, or total silence to meditate.

I don't have a good place to do it.

Any place you are can turn into a meditative spot. Trust me.

It goes against my religion.

While meditation is part of some religious practices, it has nothing to do with religion, or even spirituality (unless you want it to). More than anything else, it's about exercising your brain. Just think of it as a mental workout.

Look, if you're still feeling resistant, or are tiptoeing into Zen-ing out instead of diving in headfirst, here's a list of meditative things you can try that will still benefit you.

MEDITATIVE THINGS THAT AREN'T MEDITATION

Be aware of your emotions. I'm not asking you to stop feeling what you're feeling, but next time you feel like you're going to cry . . . or yell . . . or jump for joy . . . step outside yourself for a sec and note the emotion. If you get into the habit of doing this, you may find that you are able to de-escalate a negative emotion (like fear, anger, panic) before it gets the best of you. You can tell yourself: "I feel panicked. I feel sweaty. I feel like it's getting hard to breathe. But I don't have to go full-on attack. Let me try to take a breath or ask for help so that I can get through this quickly and without totally losing it." It's also worth noting moments when you feel calm and peaceful so that you can retrieve that feeling when you need it.

Pause while you eat. As you're eating your next snack or meal, take a moment to really taste the food. Feel it in your mouth. Chew it slowly before you swallow. Take a moment to feel grateful that you have food and that your body works well enough to process it.

Work out without music. Feel the beating of your heart instead. The breath going in and out of your body. The beads of sweat rolling down your brow. See if you can find the natural rhythm of your body. This is hard to do (at least for me) but worth a try!

Scan your body. I do this exercise in bed when I wake up or right before I go to sleep, and I find it very calming. Moving from my feet to my head, I bring awareness to each part of my body. Do my feet feel sore? My ankles wobbly? My stomach tight? I send a breath to each part of my body to relax it. And if I'm in a really generous mood, I thank my body and my organs for getting me through another big day.

Take a walk. You'd likely do this anyway, but this is a walk with intention. It's getting up from your desk, stepping outside, and taking a five-minute walk around the block . . . without your cell phone. It's finishing dinner and putting away the dishes and taking a ten-minute stroll down the street with your family . . . instead of turning on the TV. On this walk, you're going to breathe. And think a little bit. Maybe put a question in your mind and ponder the answer to it. See where your mind drifts. Maybe you'll think about your shopping list, or maybe you'll think about the breath going in and out of your body and the beat of your feet hitting the pavement. Either way, when you're done, you'll head back to your desk or your family feeling just a little more refreshed, and hopefully willing to take on any challenge.

Guess what? You're on your way to meditating.

MEDITATION FOR BEGINNERS

As I mentioned, there are all different forms of meditation. Some clear the brain. Some focus your thoughts. Some help you go deeper into yourself. A gateway form of meditation is to clear your mind by focusing on your breath. It's when you sit still in a quiet place and try to chill out your brain, dismissing active thoughts as they come into your head.

An easy way to try this is to block out five minutes of your day when you know you'll have a little privacy and quiet. I highly recommend doing this first thing in the morning before all the drama of your day starts to pile up. Find a peaceful spot without a lot of distractions. If you feel comfortable sitting on the floor in a lotus position, that's awesome; you can prop up your tush so you feel comfortable. You can also sit in a chair and rest your hands in your lap. (You're not a monk on a mountaintop, so don't let staging be an issue. You just don't want to be resting in bed or crunched up on a couch.) Now, straighten your spine and your neck and keep your shoulders down. Take a breath and close your eyes.

All you have to do is breathe. In, out. In, out. Nothing fancy. After you take a few breaths, try to pay a little more attention to your breathing. Feel the inhalations coming into your mouth, going down your throat, filling up your chest.

Now exhale . . . your lungs get smaller, the breath escapes through your nose and mouth. Bring it back in again. All you're doing is paying attention to your breath. If a thought enters your brain—*I've got to pay that bill/I forgot to buy milk/What day of the week is Christmas/Did I pack lunch for my daughter/Am I wearing matching socks/Who am I voting for in the election/Wow my butt hurts/Why don't more people of color get nominated for Oscars*—you just observe the thought and let it go. Then you get back to your breath.

Do this for five minutes. You can set an alarm or use a mindfulness app (like Insight Timer or the cleverly named Mindfulness App) on your phone so you know when to open your eyes again.

That's it. That's meditation.

The first few times you try it, it will likely feel interminable. (If five minutes really kills you, try one minute. If you can't handle one minute, try taking ten full breaths.) But like all things, the more you practice, the better you get. And like exercise, once you make meditation a part of your day, you're going to miss it when you don't have it.

People who have regular meditative practices report all the benefits I've mentioned above, or variations of it. I've also found that when you have a little more control of your brain, your thoughts, and your feelings, you don't sweat things as much. You get better at communicating. You can deal with less sleep. And when it's time to sleep, you choose it and do it. Much less tossing and turning. It's awesome.

I even got my mom on the meditation train. She found that it not only benefited her personally but it also changed the direction of what she was teaching at school. Here's what Maureen says:

I began exploring mindfulness after reading about its success with students in inner-city schools. And I could see that Beth's consistent, daily practice allowed her to maintain the stamina her work required while feeling grateful and centered in a very chaotic business. My first meditation experience was with an Oprah and Deepak Chopra twenty-one-day meditation. All of this, coupled with a blossoming yoga practice (thanks to Beth), and I was hooked! I immediately felt more peaceful and better able to handle the daily challenges of life.

Mamma Mo! I'm so proud of you!

TRANSCENDENTAL MEDITATION (TM)

Even though I'd gotten my post–plane crash anxiety under control, once I started working on *2 Broke Girls*, my panic attacks returned with a vengeance. I was spinning out from the pressure. Luckily, Whitney Cummings, the super-talented actress and comedian who is the cocreator of our show, took me aside and introduced me to a tool she used to calm her mind and body: TM, or transcendental meditation. I started to look into the practice and talked with people who did it. It turned out that without fail, the people who I admired most—those who were the most creative, most ambitious, most hardworking, and generally nicest folks around—all did TM. When I did a little more research, I discovered that Jerry Seinfeld, Jay Leno, Ellen Degeneres, and Sarah Silverman are all TM practitioners. And even though they are on the cover of magazines, they are very quiet, kind, down-to-earth, calm people.

This happened at the same time that I was getting run-down and sick, right in the middle of the skin thing. What did I have to lose? I signed up for the training and discovered that TM can help give you better workouts, lower your risk of heart disease, improve your productivity at work, aid weight loss, help build relationships, and give you a more "youthful" mind and body.

So what is this life-changing practice? Basically, it involves closing your eyes and repeating a mantra selected for you by a teacher. You start doing the meditation for a few minutes a couple of times a day and build from there. (More on why you do this on page 252.) I started doing the meditation twice a day for twenty minutes. I'd begin my morning with a session and do another at lunchtime or late in the afternoon—and always right before a taping.

TM is like working out—after a week and a half you may not see results, but after a month . . . wow. It wasn't like my brain exploded and I was dancing with the universe. But almost immediately I started noticing subtle changes. You know that afternoon slump you get—that low-energy, "I need caffeine/sugar/a pack of M&M's" feeling? Well, I noticed that if I did TM when I hit that window, the caffeine and sugar were unnecessary. I also normally had terrible road rage (inherited from Dave Behrs, thank you very much). Even when I wasn't in a hurry, I was in a hurry. That seemed to subside. When I made a full stop at a stop sign one day, Alisha and Courtney were stunned, like, "What is Beth doing?"

I quickly noticed a difference at work, too. Everything got easier—learning lines, making funny physical choices. Even eating healthy and working out were less of a struggle because I felt like all my systems were go. Plus, the fear that would engulf me when having to stay home by myself or when trying new stuff like rock climbing or paddleboarding faded away. I felt Zen. I felt calm. Totally *Point Break*, without the bank robberies.

Now I'm more in tune with my intuition than I've ever been. I'm having the best auditions of my life and finding that my acting work is the best it's been. I'm not perfect at TM (no one is), and there have been plenty of days when I've only done it once, and a few where I haven't done it at all. But when that happens, I don't beat myself up about it. I just wake up the next morning and get back to it (and usually, I can't wait to).

The great thing about TM—aside from all the amazing benefits—is that you can do it almost anywhere. You don't necessarily have to be in a dark, quiet room on a special cushion to get to the place you need to go. There's no singing bowl or gong (not that I have anything against a bowl or a gong). You can do it in the waiting room if you show up twenty minutes early for a meeting. You can do it on a plane instead of reading *US Weekly*. I have a friend that does it in the car while she's stuck in traffic. (Her husband drives. You can't drive and do TM at the same time.)

Because TM has so many fans in Hollywood, and because the details of the practice are really only shared once you sign up to make a commitment to do it, the practice sometimes gets a bad rap. It's seen as elitist or exclusive. Au contraire. The fees people pay to sign on and get trained in TM actually go toward teaching the practice to veterans suffering from PTSD, or kids in schools facing challenges like hunger or poverty. (Research by top universities and medical institutions has shown incredible benefits in educational skills for students, reduction of PTSD and depression for vets, and better coping mechanisms for abused women and girls.) My friend Alisha facilitated a TM school program. She taught in schools through the David Lynch Foundation and says that her students—who face issues like poverty and violence on a daily basis—have experienced a major change in the way they process challenges, reacting a lot more calmly and coolly during tough times.

I believe that in order to learn properly, you need to go to a proper teacher. There is a sliding fee for joining, but once you sign up, you are in for life, and you can check in whenever you need to. For the rest of your life! Just think of it as getting a degree in TM. While I was in the process of learning the practice, I read Dr. Norman Rosenthal's book *Transcendence*, where he talks to regular TM practitioners (including David Lynch, Paul McCartney, Laura Dern, and Russell Brand) about how it's changed their lives. That gave me a whole extra dimension of motivation to continue.

This is the point where you'd really like for me to explain *how* to do TM. The problem is . . . I can't. I literally signed a document saying that I wouldn't describe the process to anyone. (Everyone who signs up for TM training agrees to this.) It's not to be exclusionary, or because it's some big cult-y secret, it's just that to do TM you have to be trained correctly. It's the difference between giving your pal a massage and being trained as a massage therapist. Both feel super nice, but one is a friendly rub and the other is done with the full mental and physiological understanding of the outcome. So do yourself a favor: Go to TM.org and sign up for a free training session. If you like what you hear, and I think you will, I feel confident saying that you will never regret the pursuit of TM and the changes that it can make in your life.

I trained with a teacher named Lynn. She is the director of the David Lynch Foundation in Los Angeles, a nonprofit dedicated to providing stress-reducing TM programs to underserved and at-risk populations like inner-city students, veterans suffering from PTSD, the homeless, and abused young women and girls. I asked her to explain more about the science behind TM and why she does it as a daily practice:

> What TM is is in the name itself: *Transcend* means to go beyond, and *meditate* means to think deeply. In Transcendental Meditation we have a technique that allows the mind to effortlessly go beyond and transcend the active surface level of the mind so that one can experience the calm, peaceful area of the mind deep inside. In this state of restful alertness your brain functions with significantly greater coherence and your body gains deep rest. Rest is how our bodies are designed to balance, heal, and release stress.
>
> I learned TM as a teenager. I was looking for a natural way to relieve the stress and depression, and to find a deeper meaning to life. I experienced the reduction in the effects of stress almost right away, and the depression lifted within about eight weeks and has never returned. Thanks to TM, I've come to feel connected to my truest self and feel empowered to express who I really am.

I'm so lucky to have this amazing teacher.

MORE MINI-MEDITATIONS

If you're still looking for a way into meditation but feeling like concentration/contemplation meditation or TM aren't quite right for you yet, I'm going to recommend some of what I call "mini-meditation" practices below to get you started:

Make yourself a mantra. A mantra is a series of sounds or words that you repeat to help yourself get into a meditative state of mind. Ayurvedic doctors prescribe mantras to their patients as part of a healing process. My mom digs a mantra called Heartfulness. She repeats it to herself in her mind: "May I be peaceful, May I be healthy, May I be happy." She even uses it in her classrooms, asking her students to say the words and then send the wishes to someone else. I use one in TM that was given to me by my teacher. You can look up a mantra of your own, or use a line from a poem or a song that has a lot of resonance for you. It can just be a couple of words: Be Me. Be Free. Feel Good. Feel Peace. When in doubt, just slowly and calmly repeat a sound you may have heard in yoga class: Om.

Do guided meditation. For those of you who really like the idea of being led in meditation, seek out guided meditation—and do it for free! Go to chopra.com to be led through ten- to twenty-minute guided meditations on themes including health, creativity, and empowerment. Meditationoasis.com offers podcasts with meditations focusing on the breath, some with music and some without. (And you can make a donation if you like what you hear.) Search for "guided meditation" at yogajournal.com, and you'll find video, audio, and scripted resources for five- to fifteen-minute meditations on everything from loving kindness to eating mindfully to planning your perfect vacation (!). You can also seek out classes that offer guided meditation if you want to try a group setting.

Add intention. If you don't want to/don't have time to start your day with a full meditation sesh, you can always just set an intention, or give yourself a little mental goal to focus on throughout the day. Perch on the edge of your bed, place your feet on the ground, take a deep breath, and think about a concept or idea that you want to bring your mind back to anytime you get too caught up with the daily grind. Kindness is a great one. Or love, community, gratitude, or humility. Maybe you want to work on making a big decision, like whether you're going to take a new job or move to a new house. Maybe you want to offer a nice greeting to everyone you meet throughout the day. You could give yourself the intention to listen more and talk less. Whatever direction you want to take, plant the seed at the beginning of the day and evaluate how it went at the end.

Like a prayer. For people around the world, no matter what their faith, prayer is a super-close cousin to meditation. It's kind of like meditation directed toward someone/something/some force. So if it's a mode you feel good about, offer up your prayer in whatever form it takes . . . as long as it's not, "I pray that a tree falls on my irritating neighbor." No one/thing/force is going to sign off on that.

MAKE YOUR SPACE

If you'd like to build your practice, then creating a little meditation space in a nook or cranny of your home can help you commit to it—and feel nice and cozy while you do your mindful thing. Here's all you need to make it happen, which you probably already have at home:

A comfy chair. Some people like to sit on a pillow on the floor, or on a mat, but I suggest a comfortable chair that allows you to sit upright while supporting your back and neck. You can always use a couple of pillows to make yourself extra snug.

A soft blanket. I'm always cold, so I make sure to have a throw around me when I meditate.

Low light. You can meditate anywhere, but a room with low light (not completely dark) lets your brain chill a little better.

Mood-setters. Not required, but very helpful. Sometimes I light a candle or incense, or even make a fire in my fireplace to help set the mood.

Now, take a deep breath . . . and get your meditation on.

CHAPTER 14

GIVING BACK

Once you've done all the self-directed work we've explored in this book (eating better, moving more, getting mindful), it's time to take all the positive energy you've been manifesting and direct it toward someone else. We're talking small acts of kindness toward strangers; reassessing and recommitting yourself to important relationships in your life (even weeding out some of the toxic friendships you might be engaged in); and eventually anteing up that goodwill to lend time and effort to the causes that mean the most to you. Helping others is helping yourself. Isn't it neat how that works out?

PASSION PROJECTS

One of the most important things I learned from my family was the importance of giving back. My parents made sure that my sister and I were actively grateful for what we had in our lives, whether it was the food on our plates or the clothes in our closets. We were always super involved with our church, helping with food or toy drives, gathering clothing for the needy, or planting gardens. To this day I have many (almost too many, sometimes) charitable causes that I'm passionate about. For example, working with the ASPCA and animal rescue groups will always be a priority for me—they're how I found my way to my rescue horse, Belle. And with animals, the question is always, "Who rescued whom?"

The Rape Foundation is an organization that is also truly near and dear to my heart. One in six women is a victim of rape; one in four girls and one in six boys are sexually abused before the age of eighteen. Those are not numbers that I can live with. Luckily, organizations like The Rape Foundation make it their mission to support those who need it most by offering comprehensive care to victims of rape and sexual assault. They offer prevention programs to reduce the occurrence of these crimes and train victim service providers to enhance the help they are able to give. Gail Abarbanel is the president of the organization, and she is my hero. Hoping I could make a difference, I put together a charity run called "Sprint Away Silence" and was able to raise $25,000 for The Rape Foundation. SEE? I was able to make exercise meaningful, too.

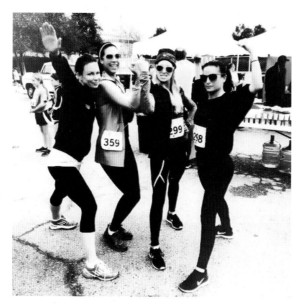

Breaking a sweat and making change for the better at the same time.

And because the arts have always done so much for me, I wanted to give back in that arena as well. It was a true stroke of luck that I landed a job at the Geffen Playhouse. Not only did it give me the opportunity to watch incredible theater, I met incredible artists, and coworkers who remain lifelong friends. I quickly saw that the Geffen's education outreach is incredible. They bring theater to children who otherwise wouldn't be able to attend a show. They also have countless other interactive outreach programs. I can't imagine not having the arts in my life, and I'm happy to support that cause as a board member.

I'm not telling you all this stuff to be like, "AHMEGAWDYOUGUYZ, aren't I just super awesome?" It's to show you that the more you do for others, the better you feel about yourself. You are contributing to karmic goodness that comes back to you in the most wonderful ways. If you are spiraling out, freaking out, worrying, stressing, consumed with your drama . . . take a deep breath. Now go do something for someone else. When you come back to your earth-shaking drama, you will find that it's really just a little kick in the dust.

How can you figure out what your passion project might be?

Start meditating. There's a reason people say they're going to "meditate" on a decision. The practice of meditation can make room in your brain for a great idea to flare up.

Time travel. Not like, in a black hole . . . I mean, reflect on your childhood and what made you feel happy as a little kid. Chances are, that childhood joy can lead you to your adult passion.

Embrace jealousy. Turn negative energy into something positive. Are you jealous of friends who always seem to have time to go to museums? Or curate vintage-jewelry connections? Or have beautiful flowers growing in their gardens? Maybe that's where your passion lies. Ask them if you can join them on their next museum visit/flea market search/trip to the greenhouse so you can start your own journey.

Find a just cause. Think about the causes that you are passionate about in the world . . . clean oceans? Animal activism? Human rights? If there's one that excites you, be it in arts, politics, or media, chances are you will find your passion play there. Do some research, offer to volunteer, show up at a rally, and get started.

Take a look. Look around your house for inspiration. What collections do you have? Ah, can't seem to let go of those Beanie Babies? Well, get proud, and start to lose yourself in the world of fellow collectors on eBay. What books are on your coffee table? If you have a lot of photo books, maybe you're a closet photographer. Pick up a camera and start to shoot. What's in your Netflix queue? If you can't stop watching *Top Gear* or other car shows, take yourself to an auto show and enjoy.

No matter what . . . don't let time or money be an object. You don't need to own sculptures; you can go to a gallery and admire them. You don't need to spearhead the entire Save the Whales campaign; you can just help with one small task. You may not be able to write a six-figure check—but maybe you have a skillset that you can offer in its place. If you're good with numbers, offer to do some accounting for an organization you like. Or if you like writing, work on some press releases or create copy for a website. And just like you do with eating well and exercising, make your passions a priority. Make a date with yourself on your calendar, and keep it.

GOING GREEN

One universal concept that everyone can get behind is going green, or making individual efforts to nurture the environment and heal the planet. This isn't just a bunch of Hollywood hoo-hah—experts agree that a little bit of effort from every city and state can alter our future for the better. You're not just me-toxing—you're detoxing the world!

Ten Easy Ways to Go Green
1. Shop at a farmers' market for your groceries. When you buy sustainably produced, local goods, you're leaving a much smaller carbon footprint.
2. Use reusable market bags (not plastic—DUH).
3. Plant a tree! Or three! Or start a garden! At my house we have lemon, orange, avocado, and fig trees, along with an herb garden, so we only need to step outside the kitchen door to spice up our lives. (I'd say "herb up our lives," but it doesn't have the same ring to it.) If you don't have access to outdoor space, try bringing a green plant into your home, planting some herbs on your windowsill, or finding a community garden you can contribute to.
4. If you're a meat eater, participate in "Meatless Mondays," or try a few days a week without meat to lessen your impact on the planet. You probably already know that lowering your meat consumption can lower your risk of heart disease, stroke, and diabetes, but it can also cut down on global water usage, greenhouse gases, and fuel dependence connected to meat production and distribution.

5. On a Saturday or Sunday, challenge yourself to walk, ride a bike, skip, rollerblade, hoverboard, whatever . . . but DO NOT use your car! Good for your body and for the environment.

6. Switch to Energy Star–rated CFL bulbs at home. It took us some getting used to because the light they shed is a little duller than our previous bulbs, but it's worth it for the positive impact on the environment.

7. Invest in a Klean Kanteen, S'well, or any other brand of reusable water bottles. I just HATE plastic water bottles. They are not only bad for the environment, they're bad for humans as well! Plastic bottles have toxins in them that can leach out after a while, and these toxins are thought to disrupt our hormonal systems and possibly lead to changes in childhood brain development.

8. Switch from heavy chemicals that can be toxic to green household cleaners. I love anything from Jessica Alba's The Honest Company. The packaging is simple and pretty, and everything smells great. And unlike some natural cleaners, they actually work really well. Best of all, they're easy to buy and keep in stock. You can do it all online and even purchase a monthly subscription.

9. Don't dump—donate! Old clothes, shoes, electronics, you name it. The landfill doesn't need them, but some lucky person will!

10. Run ONLY full loads in your dishwasher . . . if it's not a full load, just wash your dishes by hand. Why waste the water if you don't have to?

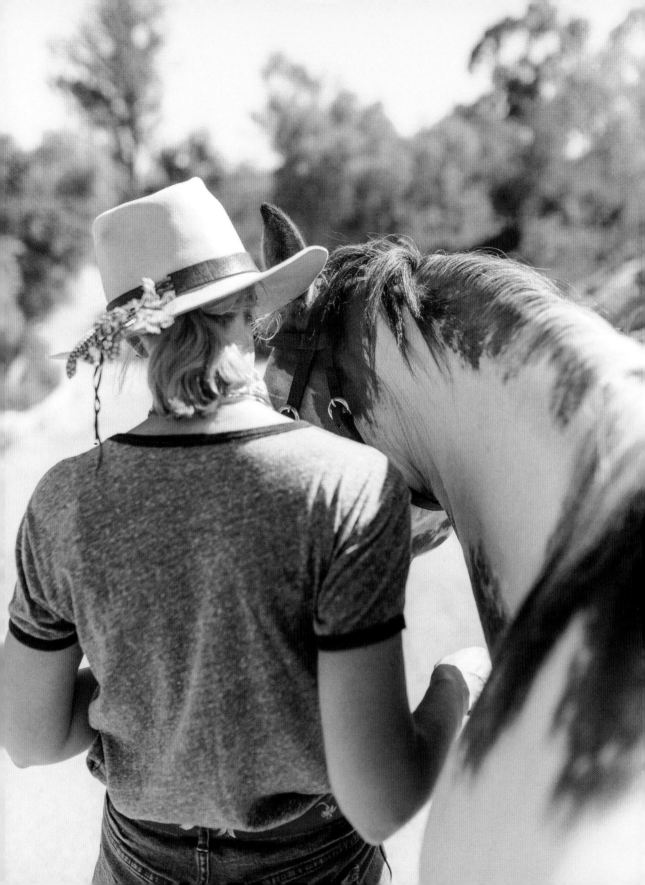

OH SO GRATEFUL . . . FOR EVERYTHING

The more mindfulness and meditative practice I brought into my life, the better things got for me. And the more aware I was that things were good. There's just this chain reaction that happens when you actively feel grateful. You start to put out the positive vibe that you feel inside. And by the law of attraction (believe it or not), that positivity comes back to you. And you will continue to thrive.

Whatever small steps you've taken to improve your life—from making yourself a smoothie, to taking a walk, to adding intention to your day (maybe all of the above?)—I know it's going to pay off for you. I often think of who I was and what I did just a few years ago. I'm really glad that I had caring people around me who called on me to take action. I'm proud of myself for committing to change yet being patient about it, knowing that long-term results take more than a hot minute. And I'm grateful to my family, friends, and coworkers for continuing to support me through the ups and downs . . . and for being willing to try some recipes along the way that WERE NOT GOOD AT ALL. I hope I can be one of those voices for you, urging you to continue when it gets tough, reminding you that instant gratification is over in, well, an instant, and believing that you can make life-long changes that will benefit your body and your mind.

I'm really grateful to you for reading this book. I hope that I've been able to help you reach your goals in changing the way you eat, move, and breathe—you know, the way you function as a human being. And doing it on your own terms. Me-toxing your body and your mind. Step by step, bit by bit, I know that we can all live healthier, happier lives.

Okay, I'm off to make a smoothie . . .

ACKNOWLEDGMENTS

I offer the deepest appreciation from the bottom of my heart to everyone who made this book possible in ways big and small, including: my family and friends, some mentioned in these pages and many more around the country; my incredible *ME-Tox* team, including Nicole Romano and Tony Lipp; Lindsay Ludwig; Bob Wallerstein; Todd Shuster and Elias Altman; Amanda Murray, Rachel Holtzman, and the staff at Weinstein Books; Taren Maroun, Dana Gallagher, Ellen Scordato, and Stonesong Press; glam girls Aviva Perea and Kindra Mann; and each and every person who contributed personal stories and testimonials to these pages. A special thank-you to Wendy Shanker—the best coauthor, pen pal, Skype date, and friend a gal could ask for. And major gratitude to my amazing fiancé, who loves me despite my being "hot pepper" challenged. Michael, I promise I will continue to keep it interesting (especially in the kitchen).

RESOURCES

ABOUT BETH

Beth Behrs
    On Twitter: @bethbehrs
    On Instagram: @bethbehrsreal

"2 Broke Girls"
    cbs.com/shows/2_broke_girls/

NUTRITION

Maya Feller, MS, RD, CDN, CLC
Maya Feller Nutrition Inc.
    mayafellernutrition.com

Jolene Hart, CHC/AADP
Beauty editor, certified health coach
and author
    jolenehart.com

Michelle Allison, RD
"The Fat Nutritionist"
    fatnutritionist.com

RECIPES

    kriscarr.com
    cookinglight.com
    rachaelray.com

ohsheglows.com
elenaspantry.com
health.com
foodnetwork.com
howsweeteats.com
marthastewart.com
blissfulbasil.com
ohladycakes.com
cestlavegan.com
elissagoodman.com
realsimple.com

WORKOUTS/YOGA

Ballet Beautiful
    balletbeautiful.com

Do Yoga with Me
    doyogawithme.com

Be More Yogic
    bemoreyogic.com

Yoga with Adriene
    yogawithadriene.com

Jessamyn Stanley
Yoga teacher and body positive activist
    jessamynstanley.com

Tara Stiles
Yoga teacher and author
  tarastiles.com

Yada Yada Yoga
  yadayoga.com

GIVING BACK

The Rape Foundation
For the support of rape treatment,
prevention, and education
  therapefoundation.org

ASPCA
American Society for the Prevention of
Cruelty to Animals
  aspca.org

Blue Apple Ranch
Inspiring responsibility and compassion
by connecting people and animals
  blueappleranch.org

Geffen Playhouse, Los Angeles
  geffenplayhouse.org

MEDITATION

Transcendental Meditation
  TM.org

David Lynch Foundation
  davidlynchfoundation.org

Dr. Norman Rosenthal
  normanrosenthal.com

The Chopra Center
  chopra.com

Meditation Oasis
  meditationoasis.com

Yoga Journal
  yogajournal.com

AND DON'T FORGET

Meghan Cleary
Shoe designer and author of *Shoe Are You?*
  shoeareyou.com

The Artist's Way: A Spiritual Path to Higher Creativity
  Juliacameronlive.com

Jessica Alba's The Honest Company
  honest.com

Vitamix
  vitamix.com

Klean Kanteen
  kleankanteen.com

S'well Bottle
  swellbottle.com

ABOUT THE AUTHORS

BETH BEHRS

Beth Behrs is one of Hollywood's most exciting actors working today. Behrs currently stars as Caroline Channing in the CBS series *2 Broke Girls* created by Michael Patrick King and Whitney Cummings. The show is one of the highest rated comedies on network television and is currently in its sixth season.

Behrs made her New York Stage Debut in Halley Feiffer's "A Funny Thing Happened on the Way to the Gynecologic Oncology Unit at Memorial Sloan Kettering Cancer Center of New York City" in the spring of 2016.

Her film credits include *Hello, My Name is Doris*, with Sally Field and Max Greenfield, and the Walt Disney Pixar animated film *Monsters University*, where she supplies the voice of Carrie Williams.

Behrs is a cocreator and cowriter of the new digital comic series called *Dents* on the LINE Webtoon platform. The project centers around a 14-year-old mutant in a post-apocalyptic future who finds herself shut out of society with superpowers she doesn't fully understand.

Behrs has performed at the Geffen Playhouse alongside Jane Lynch, Annette Bening, and Helen Mirren. She also appeared onstage with the New York Philharmonic for their New Year's Eve performance, One Singular Sensation: Celebrating Marvin Hamlisch.

In addition to singing and acting in musical theater, Behrs has been actively involved with charity organizations such as Children of the Night, American Society for Prevention of Cruelty to Animals (ASPCA), The Rape Foundation, and is a board member of the Geffen Playhouse.

WENDY SHANKER

Wendy Shanker is the author of two books: the first, a humorous, hopeful memoir about women and body image, *The Fat Girl's Guide to Life* (Bloomsbury USA), was published in nine languages around the world. Her second book, about traditional and nontraditional health, was *Are You My Guru?: How Medicine, Meditation & Madonna Saved My Life* (Penguin/NAL). Her acclaimed essay about Jewish women and body image, "Big Mouth," appeared in *The Modern Jewish Girl's Guide to Guilt*; in the recent anthology *Madonna & Me*, she tried to set Madonna up on J-Date. Her byline has also appeared in *Glamour, Self, Shape, Cosmopolitan, Teen Vogue, The Guardian UK*, and *Us Weekly* (The Fashion Police).

Wendy spent the first part of her television career working at MTV and VH1 in production, series, and specials including the VMAs and *TRL (Total Request Live)*. After a stint writing and developing women's programming at Lifetime and Oxygen, she became the head writer for major live events like *Glamour's* Woman of the Year Awards, The National Magazine Awards, and the GLAAD Media Awards, and has put words in the mouths of everyone from mega-celebs to presidents.

INDEX

Note: Page references in italics indicate photographs.

Watermelon
    buying and storing, 33
    Freeze, *145*, 146
Weight loss, 10–11, 203
Workouts. *See* Exercise

Y

Yoga
    dedication to, 216–217
    getting started with, 214–216
    health benefits from, 212–213
    mats for, 190

    poses for, 216
    psychological benefits from, 215–216
    resistance to, 213–214
    ten-minute routines, 198
Yogurt
    Dip, Spicy, 123–124
    Greek, for healing sunburns, 169
    Smooth-Out Smoothie, 44
    Spicy Indian Chicken & Spinach
        Saagwala, 111–112
    Vanilla Green Hemp Seed
        Smoothie, 45